Highs & Lows

Highs & Lows

A personal approach to living with diabetes

Michael Twist

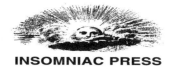

INSOMNIAC PRESS

Edited by Steven Beattie
Copy-edited by Kate Harding
Designed by Mike O'Connor

National Library of Canada Cataloguing in Publication Data

Twist, Michael, 1972–
   High & lows: a personal approach to living with diabetes

Includes index.
ISBN 1-894663-05-5

1. Twist, Michael, 1972- Health. 2. Diabetes-Patients-Canada-Biography.
I Title. II. Title: Highs and lows.

RC660.4.T85 2001   362.1'96462'0092   C2001-902144-5

The publisher and the author gratefully acknowledge the support of the Canada Council, the Ontario Arts Council and Department of Canadian Heritage through the Book Publishing Industry Development Program.

Printed and bound in Canada

Insomniac Press, 192 Spadina Avenue, Suite 403,
Toronto, Ontario, Canada, M5T 2C2
www.insomniacpress.com

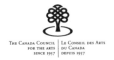

THE CANADA COUNCIL | LE CONSEIL DES ARTS
FOR THE ARTS | DU CANADA
SINCE 1957 | DEPUIS 1957

ONTARIO ARTS COUNCIL
CONSEIL DES ARTS DE L'ONTARIO

Author's Note

This book tells a personal story of living with diabetes. It was written and published from this perspective and should not be utilized as a substitute for consultation with a physician. The informational material provided herein cannot replace the insight and discernment of a professional endocrinologist. The author provides personal knowledge and experience of type 1 diabetes for illustrative purposes, but as each person with diabetes has different dietary, insulin, exercise and other requirements, this information may not be appropriate for everyone.

Dedication

This book is dedicated to the memory of Donald E. J. Black, who helped me understand I was not alone, and to all those who have diabetes.

Table of Contents

Introduction

This book is about diabetes from the inside, up close and personal, by a person who happens to have type 1, or insulin-dependent, diabetes.

There are many books about diabetes written by physicians, dieticians, psychologists and other health care professionals, which offer prescriptions and diets—this book is not like that.

It is not about exercise regimes to be followed, diabetic foot care or slick products offered by billion-dollar pharmaceutical companies selling diabetes management advances. It is also not about nonprofit organizations competing with one another in pursuit of an ever-shrinking fundraising dollar. Rather, this book is a personal response to the challenges, difficulties and experiences faced by someone living with diabetes.

When I was diagnosed with type 1 diabetes in 1989, at the age of sixteen, there was nothing to help me through my teenage frustration and grief. It was a hectic and exhausting time. Doctors offered prescriptions, nurses at the hospital illustrated injection techniques with syringes full of insulin, lab people arrived to draw my blood, and a social worker came brandishing piles of outdated information on strict diabetes management for seniors. None of this, however, could have prepared me for what I was about to take on.

Accounts of personal experiences with diabetes are sorely lacking—stories that illustrate how actual people cope with the chronic condition are few and far between. Some books that follow this path are Theresa Mclean's *Metal Jam*, Deb Butterfield's *Showdown With Diabetes*, Michael Raymond's *The Human Side of Diabetes: Beyond Doctors, Diets and Drugs*, Louise Giroux's *Taking* the Lead: Dancing with Chronic Illness, and Jerry Edelwich and Archie Brodsky's Diabetes: Caring for Your Emotions as well as Your Health. Each of these books offers a different perspective on diabetes, seeing it as more than just a physical disease that needs to be strictly managed with diet, exercise and insulin. Diabetes is a condition that involves emotions, choices, lifestyle changes, morality plays and power struggles.

This book is also about the wide gaps in the heart of conventional medicine as experienced by someone who has a chronic condition. Medicine is steeped in the acute care scientific model—performing surgery or mending broken bones—which is not always conducive to handling an ongoing medical condition with sensitivity.

Medicine also engages in a labelling process. Science has influenced our language and is intimately bound to in the way people see themselves in relation to society. Labels are simple

---

Sobering Diabetes Statistics

• One out of every twenty Canadians has diabetes (60,000 new cases are diagnosed every year). It is estimated that 2.25 million Canadians have diabetes. An additional 750,000 have type 2 diabetes, but are yet to be diagnosed. [1]

• More than 16 million Americans have diabetes. [2]

• There are approximately 135 million people with diabetes mellitus worldwide. [3]

• The World Health Organization (WHO) estimates that there will be 239 million people with diabetes in the world by the year 2010.

• Diabetes is classified as a global epidemic. [4]

• More than 75 years after the discovery of insulin, a cure for the disease has not been found, and those with insulin-dependent diabetes still must inject insulin to stay alive.

• The highest rates of type 1 diabetes recorded by the WHO in country comparisons are in Scandinavia. The U.S. and Canada have intermediate rates; Japan and Tanzania have low rates. [5]

• One in twenty women will develop diabetes during pregnancy (gestational diabetes).

and convenient to produce on demand. "Diabetic" is just such a label—it does not recognize the complexity of a person, but suggests that diabetes *is* the person. Many people forget in our fast-paced, scientific world that there is a person before the disorder; this book is about a person. Crucially, I am not a diabetic—I am a person with diabetes. I would more likely call myself a writer, inline skater, hockey player, musician or even a human being rather than a "diabetic." Yes, diabetes is part of me, but it's not all of who I am.

This book discusses the many misconceptions that plague those with diabetes; misconceptions that are all too often based on old information, rumours and false stereotypes. Employers still fear that people with diabetes are a liability in the workplace, a hazard in a position of responsibility, or simply people who take a lot of sick days. Employers still actively exclude people with diabetes from their workforce, regardless of the facts. Even the government imposes blanket restrictions on the diabetes population in areas such as vehicle licensing and military eligibility. The reality of discrimination that people with diabetes experience throughout their

---

• In Canada, the economic burden of diabetes was estimated at over $13 billion Canadian annually, which is roughly $9 billion U.S. This estimate is based on a Canadian population that is one-tenth the size of the American population. [6]

• In 1998, 16 million people in the U.S. alone had diabetes, which is up 700 percent since 1959, compared to 750,000 who had HIV/AIDS, 4 million who had Alzheimer's and 8 million who had cancer. More than 180,000 people die annually from diabetes, compared to 50,000 annually from AIDS. The economic and social costs of diabetes were $98.2 billion U.S. in 1998. The National Institutes of Health, despite these figures, funded approximately $2 billion U.S. for AIDS research, $3 billion U.S. for cancer research and only $376 million U.S. for diabetes. [7]

• According to Diabetes UK (formerly the British Diabetic Association), over 1.4 million people in the U.K. have diabetes.

lives is, like most other forms of discrimination, based on ignorance.

Diabetes is often misunderstood, because it comprises a wide range of conditions that may require a variety of treatments. Definitions of diabetes as they currently exist in medicine are problematic. Diabetes is not one illness—it's different things to different people.

Diabetes has not been cured. Insulin, while one of the most significant medical discoveries of the twentieth century, is not a cure—it only helps control the chronic condition. People with insulin-dependent diabetes are often forced to juggle the daily tasks of blood tests, insulin injections, a diet and an exercise schedule along with the highs and lows of everyday life. They are often young and healthy individuals who are attempting to live with diabetes beyond the diagnosis.

People whose lives are touched by diabetes, such as health care professionals and parents of children who have diabetes, also have crucial roles to play in changing public perceptions of diabetes. Reading this book will give valuable insight into the complexities of managing the physical and emotional aspects of

---

Diabetes accounted for 9 percent of the annual National Health Service (NHS) budget in 2000. This amounts to a staggering £4.9 billion, roughly $10.5 billion Canadian.
• Diabetes and its complications kill more people annually than breast cancer, AIDS, and lupus combined. Diabetes is the single most frequent reason for physician visits, use of hospital outpatient facilities and hospitalization. Fewer than 5 percent of Canadian medical research dollars are devoted to diabetes research. During their lifetimes, many people with diabetes may experience blindness, nerve damage, stroke, amputation or kidney disease, even though they inject insulin to control their blood sugar levels.

the condition, which are in a constant state of flux.

Please note that I am by no means a qualified medical professional. There are many books out there by medical professionals who do not live with diabetes every day of their life. I admit I'm no Ph.D. or MD. I have a humble BA in communications from Simon Fraser University. I am a person with diabetes who has lived with the condition for over twelve years and has something to say about it. I hope that this book will provide newly diagnosed patients with what I did not have—not a prescription, information brochure or a medical textbook, but a book that tells a personal story.

My goal is to illustrate what diabetes is like for a person who actually experiences it daily, and to promote awareness of diabetes as a serious chronic condition.

Part One
MY STORY

Chapter 1
Diabetes 101

Different Strokes for Different Folks

There are three main flavours of diabetes: type 1 (insulin-dependent, or "juvenile"), type 2 (non-insulin-dependent, or "adult-onset") and type 3 (gestational diabetes). All are called diabetes because of their relation to the pancreas—the long, thin organ located behind your stomach. The pancreas plays a key part in the digestive process and metabolism, as it regulates sugar in the blood by secreting insulin (which lets cells change sugar into energy, which lowers blood sugar); glucagon (which breaks down a substance in the liver, known as glycogen, to raise blood sugar); and somatostatin (which regulates the production and release of both insulin and glucagon). This process is not clearly understood, as there are many hormones and complex functions within an individual that make things like blood sugar levels difficult to predict. But we'll get into that later.

Diabetes is not a simple equation of insulin and food. The pancreas produces insulin, but that is only a small part of its function as a digestive organ. The pancreas is involved in a strange sort of balancing act, trying to deal with whatever the body eats (because all food is broken down into sugar eventually, unless it's stored as fat) and produce substances that allow the body to function. These substances keep blood sugar balanced—not too high and not too low.

People who have type 1 diabetes must take daily injections of insulin to survive and most likely have a pancreas that produces no insulin at all. Without insulin, the sugar hangs around in the blood stream, unable to enter the cells to produce energy, and therefore produces high blood sugar.

Type 1 diabetes used to be called "juvenile" because it usually occurs in people under 30 years of age, although it can occur at any time during a person's life. It is caused when the immune system attacks the beta cells of the pancreas, which produce insulin. What is not known is why the immune system kicks into hyperdrive and attacks its own body.

There is no known relationship between type 1 diabetes and climate, seasons, consumption of sugar or physical trauma. It is, however, linked to genetic susceptibility; in other words, if it's in your family, you're more likely to have it. Medicine is baffled as to what triggers diabetes—it has been variously suggested that a virus, metabolic stress and adolescence may all have some role to play.

Type 2 usually occurs in people over 40 years of age, hence the term "adult-onset," and is usually hereditary and related to obesity. The pancreas does not produce enough insulin, or uses it ineffectively. People with type 2 diabetes may be able to control their condition with diet, excerise and/or medications, but some

---

Diabetes Symptoms

All of the following symptoms are used to diagnose diabetes. If you have any of the following persistent and unexplainable symptoms, visit your physician.

- Frequent urination
- Excessive thirst
- Weight loss
- Weakness
- Drowsiness
- Abdominal pain
- Vomiting
- Fruity-smelling breath

will also require insulin injections.

Type 3, or gestational diabetes, is a temporary condition that occurs during pregnancy, but it creates an increased risk of developing type 1 or 2 diabetes for both mother and child later in life.

You would think the differences between types 1, 2 and 3 would be easy to understand, but they're not. Type 1 can occur at any age, so Grandpa may have "juvenile diabetes." Type 2 is now an epidemic among young Native populations in Canada, which many believe to be caused by obesity and changing diets. Gestational diabetes (type 3) is transitional, developing during pregnancy and disappearing after the baby is born. It's not a lifetime condition like type 1, or a progressive condition like type 2.

Diabetes plagues the young and old. People with type 1 are the minority, comprising about 10 percent of all people with diabetes, while type 2 accounts for the other 90 percent of North Americans that have diabetes. Some 6.5 percent of women who had children under two years of age in 1995 reported gestational diabetes in their most recent pregnancy.

The term "diabetic" is often used to describe both a child with type 1 diabetes who must inject insulin on a daily basis and a senior citizen who must take pills and follow a diet. This is one of the main difficulties in defining the condition, and it can contribute to misconceptions.

Risk Factors for Diabetes [8]
For type 1 (insulin-dependent) diabetes:
  • Race and ethnicity (specifically people of Aboriginal, African, and Latin American descent)
  • A family history of diabetes
  • Exposure to an environmental trigger such as an unidentified virus (thought to stimulate an immune system attack against the beta cells of the pancreas)

For type 2 (non-insulin-dependent) diabetes:
  • A family history of diabetes

Without complicating the matter further, we must learn to open our mind to the multi-faceted nature of this chronic condition and be careful not to assume that all people with diabetes are old, fat and ate too much candy when they were kids. These misconceptions only serve to create fears and ignorance, and make people with diabetes want to tear out their hair in frustration.

Watch Your Language
The full medical term for diabetes is "diabetes mellitus." The term "diabetes" is derived from the Greek word *dia* (meaning "through") and *betes* (meaning "go"). The term originally came from the idea of a siphon—as if the body was siphoning water, producing symptoms of excessive thirst and urination.

Mellitus is the Latin word for honey, and was added in the seventeenth century because of a rather disgusting way to diagnose a patient—by tasting his or her urine, which would be sweet. Thankfully, doctors today are a little less intimate with their patients. Even if they ask you for a urine sample, odds are they won't use it for this purpose.

The words "disease," "disorder," "illness" and "chronic," although some are used in this book, all have negative baggage attached to them and are imperfect words to describe diabetes.

Even the words "cure," "health" and "medicine" have their

• Age (usually over 40 years old)
• Obesity
• Sedentary lifestyle
• Race and ethnicity (specifically people of Aboriginal, African, and Latin American descent)
• A previous diagnosis of impaired glucose tolerance

For type 3 (gestational) diabetes:
• A larger than average baby

own biases. The word "health," for example, is based on the Anglo-Saxon word *hale* meaning "whole." Health therefore implies wholeness. If health means being whole then what does that suggest for people with diabetes? Can you achieve perfect health when you're managing a chronic condition? For that matter, can anybody achieve perfect health? Well-being might be a better term to use, because it includes both mental and physical soundness for a person, rather than implying that to be healthy, you must be whole. People who are blind or who are missing a limb can still be well.

The word "medicine" is based on the Latin root *mederi* meaning "to cure," and also on the root meaning "to measure." The notion of practicing "medicine" to treat a chronic condition reveals the problems inherent in the language.

Applying a label such as "diabetic" to someone and then walking away is not very useful, but scientists love to apply labels to everything from chemical compounds to animals and humans. Since diabetes is such a complex condition, the application of one blanket label to all those who live with it is reductionist and exclusive.

The word "normal" suggests two things: 1) typical, usual, average or ordinary, and 2) healthy in mind and body. I think I've always had problems with this word because of the treatment recommendations from medical professionals: Your blood sugar should be "normal"; your Hemoglobin A1c (a blood test that attempts to assess blood sugar control over time) should be "normal." Don't get drawn into thinking of yourself as abnormal if you have diabetes.

I am calling attention to the meaning of these words to highlight the perspective on the world that they imply. As the physicist David Bohm points out, the idea of health is "regarded as the outcome of a state of right inward measure in all parts and processes of the body."[9] Measurement is what science is all about. Measure Hemoglobin A1cs, test blood sugars and adjust insulin dosages all you like, but the fact remains that diabetes has not been cured and is a chronic condition—the treatment of which is not surprisingly geared toward by the idea of measurement in the hands of conventional medicine.

Measurement implies control in following a schedule or regimen. The ability to measure blood sugar, insulin dosages, Hemoglobin A1c, food carbohydrate content and urine ketone levels will not cure diabetes. Such ability may make the patient feel as though she is more in control, but this control comes at a price. An obsession with measurement will impede the day-to-day quality of life that a person with diabetes experiences.

Moreover, medical science remains mired in an obsession with measurement, despite the inability of many medical professionals to agree upon the implications of such measurement. For example, a Hemoglobin A1c result may be too high for one physician, while for another it may be perfectly normal. Or a patient's insulin dosages may be lowered in a hospital environment in order to keep blood sugar high, despite regular blood sugar readings that suggest the patient needs more insulin to maintain a normal level in an inactive environment.

Diabetes is a good introduction to the limitations of words, since it's often difficult to find the right words to describe the many aspects of this condition. In this book I am sensitive to words because I know their power, and rather than fall into the conventional trap of calling people with diabetes "diabetics," as many books on the subject do, I want to emphasize the person behind the label.

Chapter 2
My Diabetes Diagnosis

Diagnosis Day (D-Day)

I did not have the faintest idea what diabetes was going to do to my life. I had read in the booklet Dr. James gave me that once you had it, you had it for life, but that could be true of a runny nose, and I did not take it too seriously. I did not understand then that it was not just a life condition, but also a life sentence. [10]

Theresa Mclean likens the diagnosis of diabetes to a prison sentence. She committed no crime, but she was condemned to life with diabetes without parole. Good behaviour wouldn't necessarily mean no complications, either. She did not realize the full impact of the chronic condition at the outset—something that had an impact on her entire life.

My own D-Day fell on March 4, 1989, just days away from my seventeenth birthday. That day I was admitted into Langley Memorial Hospital, even though I felt fine. My age presented a bit of a paradox: I was old enough to learn diabetes management, but young enough to visit the Children's Hospital outpatient clinic.

In terms of diagnosis horror stories, I have none. There are people who undergo a life-threatening incident, such as collapsing during basketball or keeling over at a party, because their body is starved for energy even though there's excess sugar in their blood. (Without insulin, the sugar in the bloodstream cannot enter cells to produce energy.) I do remember basketball practice; running up and down the court thinking I was going to die, my cells starving for sugar. I was unbelievably thirsty, as if I had been travelling in the desert for hours—a thirst so intense I could literally drink a pitcher full of water at one sitting. Water flushes out the excess sugar from the bloodstream, which explains the ensuing symptom of frequent urination. The drinking fountain was my newfound oasis, and the bathroom my second home. My pancreas had kicked the insulin bucket. It was then that I realized I was sick and I needed a doctor.

I still remember the message on the answering machine from my family doctor, matter-of-factly stating that my blood sugar was 42 millimoles per litre and that I should go to the hospital immediately. A normal blood sugar, I was soon to learn, is within the ideal boundaries of 4 and 8 millimoles per litre (75–150 milligrams per decilitre).

My initial feeling was shock as my parents checked me into Langley Memorial Hospital. The only other time I'd been in a hospital was as a child, when I'd fallen off a train in a playground and split my head open, requiring stitches. But this was something different altogether—the cut on my head healed, but diabetes would not.

My mother, a social worker, denied it from the start. Even when I was showing all the classic symptoms: weight loss, excessive thirst, frequent urination, fatigue and nausea. She ignored it, but why shouldn't she? Why would she want to admit that her child had a chronic condition? My dad didn't say much. I can hardly imagine the horror my parents felt at the moment I was diagnosed. As Mclean wrote, it sounded like a sentencing: You are now condemned to live with a chronic condition for the rest of your life. Do not pass go; do not collect $200.

During my hospital stay, insulin shots were prescribed to bring my soaring blood sugar down to normal range. When it came down, I developed all the other symptoms the doctor told me I would—especially blurred vision, which lasted for a few days.

In the hospital I experienced my first real taste of information overload. Future university assignments paled in comparison to the excruciatingly boring and seemingly useless information I was expected to read. It clogged my brain cells and generated misinformed worries—unfounded delusions like that I was going to die of this rare and strange illness, that I would catch some other illness in the hospital, that nobody in the world had diabetes but me, and that I had instantly become an alien on a planet known as high school. At that time in my life I wanted nothing that would set me apart as an outcast.

I held a faint hope that the Canadian Diabetes Association (CDA) information might prove useful to me in the future. However, the information was horribly out of date at the time I received it and is completely useless now. The information was directed at the stereotypical person with diabetes—the two-dimensional caricature that finds its way into much hollow diabetes-related literature intended for seniors—and bore little resemblance to the person I was at the time. The information was sadly inadequate and did not apply to me personally. I needed something to fill in the missing gaps.

I was sixteen, going on seventeen, and it seemed to me that most of the information for those with diabetes was not exactly appropriate for my age group. My feelings of isolation and grief were pronounced.

To counteract these feelings of profound alienation, I began a diary in the hospital as a form of catharsis. What follows is my hospital experience, almost verbatim.

The Hospital Experience
I wake up alone, drowsily clutching the pillow of the hospital bed and hoping it has all been a bad dream. I am the only teen on the pediatric ward.

As some kid starts singing "Jingle Bells" down the hallway, an eerie feeling creeps over me. I feel the fear of a child, singing as a way to summon up the mythical comfort that a Christmas song brings. He sings the song because it somehow numbs his pain.

Jingle bells, jingle bells
Jingle all the way...

I want to tell the kid to shut up. No one should be subjected to this kind of abuse while trying to sleep. But hospitals are always like that. I'll be lucky if the kid next to me doesn't snore or the one in the body cast doesn't call for the nurse in the middle of the night, complaining. It's almost impossible to sleep in a hospital at the best of times, let alone when a kid is singing Christmas carols in March.

Aren't hospitals supposed to cure you of illness and take away the pain? That's what doctors are supposed to do, right? Take away the illness, operate, prescribe pills, so that people can continue their healthy lives. Illness as the enemy of life must be operated on and destroyed. These doctors are like digital shamans with their veil of objectivity and pharmacies full of magically potent potions.

Hospitals are not places for children, or anybody, for that matter. The green-clad apparitions with cold hands arrive in the night and frequently reach into cribs for another test. More lab work needs to be done, all in the name of science and doctor's liability, and parents try to calm their horrified children. A cure will come, surely, because no God would ever allow this suffering to continue.

The song stops abruptly as I sit up in the hospital bed, my mind racing non-stop. A sound in the night stirs me awake and I struggle to hear it again in the silence. I wonder what happened to the kid.

Now it's early morning. I fall back into the bed and pretend that I'm sleeping. It's easier than facing breakfast and the events that now go with it.

My room is tiny, with only one window gracing the wall to the left of my bed. The curtains that hang over it give the colourful impression of vomit, and they block out the sun—hardly inspiring those imprisoned inside to get any better.

What will I do for the rest of the day after breakfast? Watch television? Wonder why senior citizens and kids are on the same ward in some strange blurring of childhood and adulthood? Say hello to my geriatric neighbours? Ponder the cruel joke that's being played out?

The nurse makes noise busily as she ensures I'm awake. She has a syringe and some bottles that she places on my bedside table, as if they are naturally part of the scenery and not worth mentioning.

"How was your sleep?"

"Jingle bells, jingle bells…"

"That was Samuel. He's in here because he has a liver infection."

"Poor kid."

She draws the insulin from a tiny bottle into the syringe and rubs alcohol on my arm.

"Better get used to it," she says, as she jabs it into my arm.

"What?"

"You're going to have to learn how to do this. A nurse can't inject your shot all the time."

I like her, even though she is trying to rush me into my fate. Besides, she is just doing her job. Nobody around here has any time, and any that is left is reserved for the kids, not a teenager like me. In that way I am like an adult, and I could go and watch the TV in the geriatric ward any time I want.

Breakfast comes in a plastic tray arranged in sections to be sure each portion doesn't mix with the surrounding food. Hospital food has a suspicious consistency somewhat like baby food. I decide to eat it because I'm so hungry. Luckily, I am allowed the privilege of choosing my own restricted menu. These are menus they give special people who can't have excessive doses of sugar. It seems glucophobia is running rampant through diabetes education. I know that everything you eat is broken down into sugar, except fat, so taking sugar out of your diet is technically impossible.

I veer away from the sausages and the other "questionable ingredient" dishes and choose less ambiguous food, like cheese sandwiches, cookies and fruit, which are more appealing. I also plan to visit the local corner store for a chocolate bar as soon as the nurse isn't watching me—something they call "cheating" on your diet, as if it was some covert operation, a moralistic choice. Maybe if I follow my diet, take insulin and do blood tests like I'm supposed to, they'll let me go to heaven. The argument for this impossible diet is the prevention of complications later in life; but even a strict diet and immaculate blood sugar control will not guarantee the absence of complications. It is a roll of the genetic dice.

Time passes slowly in the hospital, so I am euphoric whenever a friend visits. Some girl passes by the doorway to my room, pushing a cart. Startled, I suddenly I feel self-conscious in my one-size-fits-all hospital pajamas, and I pull up the bed covers to hide them.

"Hi," Jessica says, seeing me pull up the covers.

"Hey. How're you doing?"

"Fine, though this place is kind of freaky," Jessica remarks.

"Yeah, tell me about it. Boring as hell."

"What are you in for?"

I think of lying, but the embarrassing word comes to my lips. "Diabetes."

"Diabetes? I thought only old people get that."

"No, anyone can get it."

"You don't look like there's anything wrong with you. It's not contagious or anything, is it?" Jessica covers her face half-jokingly and starts to back up.

"Funny. Do you think they'd keep me in here with these other people if I was contagious?"

"So when are you out?"

"Soon, I hope. You work here?"

"Work experience from school."

"I see. Having fun?"

"Overjoyed. Want to go for a walk?"

"Sure. If I can get changed first."

Jessica smiles and I think that maybe the hospital isn't so bad after all. She takes me away as if I didn't have an illness anymore.

It crosses my mind that I could just leave with her and go see a movie or something, no questions asked. But diabetes is there, right in my face. She sees my troubled expression and hollowed eye sockets from my weight loss.

Jessica walks me back and writes her phone number on my book. I think maybe something good can come out of this unexpected hospital visit, and I decide to call her when I escape.

The next day my parents visit, bringing their gifts of diet pop and books. It's some strange-tasting diet pop they bought down in the States. Never before had I appreciated that which was sugar-free.

My parents are probably more scared that I am—I can tell by their faces and by the way they talk to me like I was a kid again. I thank them and ask for a magnifying glass so that I can read the books they bring me; my body had adapted to the excessively high blood sugar, and bringing it back down to normal has resulted in temporary blurred vision. After my parents leave, Dan from school comes to visit. It's great to see him.

"So you're a diabetic?" Dan asks.

"Yeah, that's what they say."

"My great-grandfather was a diabetic."

"Oh."

"He couldn't have any sugar and had to boil his needles."

"Well, now it's plastic syringes. And they blood-test now."

"Blood test? Doesn't it hurt?"

"Haven't done it yet."

Dan thinks for a while, taking in the décor.

"You didn't miss anything. School sucks."

"That bad, huh?"

"I won't elaborate."

Dan produces my homework from his bag.

"You shouldn't have. No really, you shouldn't have. Can't you take it back and say I'm unconscious?"

"Nice try. What's up with you?"

"Nothing much. I'm alive. This diabetes thing should be over soon. Doctor said after they bring my blood sugar down and get me under control I can go home."

"Good."

He knows I'm lying. Diabetes has no quick cure. I'll be a person with diabetes for the rest of my life.

I walk Dan down to the front doors and tell him about Jessica, and then I watch him leave.

The emergency area is dead quiet and visiting hours are over. I wander back to the room and find the nurse waiting.

"Where have you been?" she asks.

"I went for a walk."

She stands beside me, loading her syringe with the tiny bottles of liquid. The needle finds its destination in my arm. It isn't nearly as bad as the blood work they took when I first came in.

After dinner, which might have made me ill again, Dr. Bacchus shuffles in.

"Anybody talked to you about what's going on?"

"No, not really."

Bacchus sighs and swallows hard, trying to look serious.

"Your pancreas has stopped producing insulin, which is a hormone that breaks down the food you eat and changes it into glucose for your body to use as energy. The medical term for this condition is diabetes mellitus, and there is currently no cure for it. It can be controlled by insulin injections. I'm putting you on two injections a day with regular and NPH insulins to regulate your blood sugar. Fluctuations are unhealthy, so you'll need to follow a diet. High doses of sugar, such as in candy or regular pop, should be avoided because they will raise your blood sugar too quickly. High blood sugar is called hyperglycemia and low blood sugar is called hypoglycemia..."

He lost me long ago, probably about the time he left the deadpan message on my answering machine telling me to come to the hospital. He stares at me now, searching my face for a clue, and gets up—I'm hard to read. He writes some notes on my chart then quickly leaves to catch the elevator. I look over at the pile of information I am supposed to read. Thank you for the textbook reading. Can I talk to a human being now?

Linda is human. She is a social worker and she is assigned to me, to help me along with my first injection. I am not ready, but who would be?

I suddenly lament the passing of my former existence. The time I could eat and drink freely, whatever I wanted. Maybe a little tired, thirsty, urinating a lot, but was that so bad compared to taking injections every day? I had also lost a bit of weight—going from 175 pounds down to 140 in the course of a couple months—but that wasn't as bad as this.

My stocking feet take me down the hallway, past the elevators and the nurse's station and the geriatric ward to the TV room.

I hear an old man gargle, or it might be a cough. An elderly woman calls for a nurse. I sit in the TV room enjoying relative isolation, because all the old-timers have been put to bed. I look outside the window into the darkness of the trees and the moon in the pitch-black sky.

Flipping through the channels to kill the boredom, I avoid my hospital room because of the events that are part of it. I decide finally that I need to stay, because I cannot run from diabetes, no matter how much I feel I could escape. I am simultaneously sad and angry.

TV takes away these thoughts briefly. I drink coffee, because it's there, and dump artificial sweetener in it. I hate its acrid taste, but sugar is off limits.

I walk back to my room, enjoying the relative freedom of an adult. I am dead tired anyway, looking at the time that has slipped away. I pull the clean covers back and slip into bed. Sleep pulls me away.

I fall through the immense sky, plummeting as the wind rushes through my hair, ringing in my ears. I hear sleigh bells.

...Oh what fun it is to ride
In a one horse open sleigh,
Hey!

I feel pacified. As if everything is all right, even in the face of immense danger. Then, without warning, the earth becomes larger and larger and I begin to spin wildly out of control. Fear suddenly wraps around me like a faulty parachute. Faster and faster the ground becomes larger and I scream into the deafening wind.

I awake with a start, lying in the hospital bed, soaked in cold sweat. I can barely think. I raise my leaden arm to press the little red button that seems miles away on the railing beside my bed. White coats fly past me like angels' wings. I hallucinate a hazy heaven, feeling a yearning hunger in my stomach. My tongue and lips are numb and the White Coats are putting something into my arm.

I soon learn that I can't trust diabetes. Predictability is thrown out the window—the diet and the tests all serve to lessen the unpredictable factors and risks to existence. The nurse enters.

"Good morning, time for a blood test."

Does she expect me to jump up all excited, like a hospitalized Julie Andrews with a song coming on? The hills aren't exactly alive with the sound of music.

"You had an insulin reaction last night."

"Yeah. Insulin does that?"

"Insulin controls the blood sugar, but you can still go high or low. You went low."

She places the plastic machine before me and teaches me how to load the penlike device with a needle-sharp lancet. I apprehensively apply it to the end of my finger. I push the button and it quickly stabs a hole in my finger. Blood forms and I squeeze a bead carefully onto a thin plastic strip and wait. The machine counts down. It reminds me of a bomb, electronic countdown and all. I wipe it with a tissue when it beeps some more, then wait again; this perpetual waiting I will learn to dread. The result is displayed with a series of more beeps. I am 13 millimoles per litre; I am a number—and a bit high. She takes out the lancet with her gloved hands and drops it into the biological waste container.

"Very good. That result's much better than the 42 you were when you came in."

"What's the normal range?"

"Between four and eight, roughly."

I feel as if I've failed, as if someone with a "normally" functioning pancreas was somehow morally better than me. The two insulin bottles clank together as she brings them up to the light and draws insulin into the syringe. She hands it to me.

"I'd like you to try it yourself today."

"Me? Aren't you supposed to do it?"

"Well, you might as well. It'll give you practice."

I con my way out by promising that I'll do it tomorrow morning before breakfast.

"Tomorrow with Linda? That's a deal?" she asks.

"Yeah."

She sticks it into the fleshy part of my arm behind my muscle. "Was that so bad?"

I don't answer as she leaves and I adjust my one-size-fits-all pajamas before wandering out of the stuffy room to roam the hallways like a ghost.

These hospital days crawl by slothlike, as a stream of diabetes information accumulates beside my hospital bed. Dieticians, nurses, lab people and the doctor all come to see me, each with a pile of pamphlets and endless lectures.

I awake one morning, groggily realizing there is something foreign in my arm that is burning. I look up to find someone standing beside me with gloved hands. Crimson fluid is being sucked out of me into a huge needle much larger than my insulin needles. I groan in pain and think of vampires, feeling my arm deflate. I feel as if I might faint, even though I am lying down.

"There. All done," Vampire Woman from the lab says, "I didn't want to wake you."

How thoughtful. She holds five tubes of my blood in her rubber hand. I only saw one being filled. After leaving a piece of cotton on the bite, she leaves the room, carrying her kit full of goodies. I've been violated, as if I was an unfeeling corpse.

I get up and walk to the window, brushing the curtains aside to let the sun pour in on me and my no-name pajamas. Linda suddenly comes in.

"It's insulin time...and your turn today."

I consider jumping out the window, but that would only delay the inevitable.

I go back to the bed and sit on the edge, with a sickening feeling in my stomach. I stare at the wall as I take the two bottles and a syringe from her. First the regular insulin then the NPH, so as not to contaminate the clear regular insulin with the milky NPH's long-acting drug. Makes for fewer blood sugar fluctuations to combine them at dose time. "Is this right?" I keep asking her. She reassures me that I'm doing fine. Of course it's not fine or natural that I'm injecting a foreign substance into my body, but the method is sound.

The syringe is full. I decide to do it in my leg. No problem. Just slip it in and push down the plunger, right? I aim the loaded needle at the mound of skin on my leg, but each time I try to puncture it, I bring it back. Then my hand starts to tremble—I realize again that I can't do it.

I have no choice; it is a matter of survival. But no matter how much I try to rationalize sticking a syringe into my body, the harder it becomes. It's like a plastic bandage that is stuck on a wound, and taking it off will bring a scab with it. Either it comes off slowly and painfully, or it is pulled off quickly. With the nurse looking on eagerly, it is even more difficult—but she has to be sure that I will take it.

There is no point in delaying the inevitable any further. There is no turning back. The needle is in and the insulin is gone, slowly absorbing into my bloodstream. Though it didn't hurt at all, the tears come unrestrained, the floodgates open, the room begins to cave in on itself. There is no denying it—diabetes is a part of me from this moment on. All the learning and preparation in the world could not have made me ready to inject myself with a syringe full of insulin. Psychologically, it is far more difficult than pricking my finger for blood tests.

My parents and grandparents visit later that day. Other friends and family visit to cheer me up, though I don't *look* sick anymore, having slowly gained back some of the weight I'd lost. I want to go home, even though I am still frightened about what that means—I will have an unwelcome companion with me. Diabetes is something deep inside, with no recognizable outward appearance. Should I keep it all a secret?

The hospital was my home until March 15, 1989. Days that dragged on forever, full of useless and wrong-headed information. The pamphlets I was given included typical fodder such as "Aiming for Good Control in Diabetes," "Metric Measures" and "Eating Plans and Menus." These tracts obsessed over measurement and the importance of controlling the diabetes condition, while others were more psychologically focused, such as the pithy "Looking Up Is Better than Feeling Down."

This "uplifting" pamphlet read, in part: "The diabetes way of living is not a 'normal' lifestyle." Thanks for pointing that out right after my diagnosis. There are plenty of other sadistic platitudes contained in the pamphlet, including this gem: "You can and must take charge of your diabetes. How does that make you feel? Hopefully you will see this as a challenge." Sorry, but it's not entirely uplifting to someone recently diagnosed with a chronic condition to have to digest this kind of information. In fact, it's liable to make you "feel down."

Quick quiz. What's wrong with the following: "...diabetes means changing certain lifelong habits, enforcing restrictions and making scheduling changes. All of these take time to accept—from several months to a year or two." First, at sixteen, I hadn't quite developed lifelong habits. Second, imagine the self-criticism that could hound a person with diabetes who reads that they should get over being diagnosed and accept all of the restrictions and scheduling challenges that accompany this diagnosis within a maximum of two years. It's been much more than two years for me, and I still haven't accepted it. I don't think I ever will. Diabetes isn't acceptable at all, and I don't think that people with diabetes should be forced to "accept" the condition, or to "comply" with treatment. There's a big difference between adjusting to something and accepting it, and between complying with and adhering to a new set of rules.

In the hospital, I was taught to swab the injection site with alcohol, to cleanse the area of bacteria. They taught me also to swab before pricking my finger for a blood test or injecting insulin. This toughens the skin over time, so it's teaching I've since dispensed with. I also re-use syringes and lancets, because I feel that using them only once and throwing them away is a waste. Pincushion fingers and bruised injection sites are the stories of my life, and sometimes I need to break the rules.

I have been injecting insulin twice a day, sometimes more, ever since I bridged the psychological gap that fateful day in the hospital. According to the doctor, if I don't inject insulin, I'll die within a few days. I figure it is probably a good idea to take insulin.

Diabetes is there like a monkey on my back, a strange parasite that stays with me, forever asserting itself at the most inopportune times, forever bringing my feet back down to Earth.

Chapter 3
The Aftermath

Back to School

I never did like high school. My memories are of cliques, posing, designer jeans, fights, crappy food, boring classes and lame dances. As much as I disliked high school, however, it was a learning experience I had to endure to become who I am today.

Diabetes made high school that much harder because I didn't know anybody else who had it. I felt like I was the only one in the universe who had diabetes. I kept it largely hidden from my classmates, and only my close friends knew I had it. I played on the basketball team and never heard the end of people asking me if I would try out for rugby, which I never did—not because of my diabetes, but because I was not keen on breaking my neck.

I would compensate during basketball by having a snack before a game, which wouldn't help much if I sat on the bench, which I did a lot. If I got low, it would usually be after a practice because our coach ran us hard.

The coach never made an exception because of diabetes. He knew, but not many others on the team did. I thought at the time if the other players knew, they would have treated me differently, and I believe now that they probably would have. I guess it was the high school pressure of having to pretend you're like everybody else. I already knew that I wasn't like everyone else—not everyone is 6-feet-6-inches tall—and diabetes wasn't something I'd volunteer to tell everybody.

I never made a fuss about diabetes in school. I never broadcasted it because I didn't want to be treated differently. I didn't want my peers to tiptoe around me at parties, or be afraid to offer me a can of pop, or ask too many prying questions. I wasn't sure anybody would understand. Many friends hardly knew I had it. In fact, everything seemed back to normal in their eyes, but it wasn't normal at all for me.

As for insulin reactions at school, I had a few, but never lost consciousness. I knew when they were coming and what had to be done to counteract them—eat sugar and wait. It was, and it still is, the waiting game that is the most difficult aspect. You get low, you eat something to get back to ideal blood sugar, and then you have to wait with that horrible shaky, weak feeling. Gradually, everything is back to normal again, it's as if the fact of hypoglycemia had been a hallucination.

I always rode my bike home from school in the years before I got a beat-up Toyota. My mom would drop me off in the morning and I'd brave the Langley traffic on the ride home through the countryside. It was not the greatest idea in the winter, but it probably contributed to my current love of bicycles. Not once did I run into trouble because of diabetes, despite riding home almost every day.

I remember having to eat morning and afternoon snacks, which I eventually cut out myself, and waking up early on weekends to inject my insulin in the morning, then eating a full breakfast before going back to bed (and sometimes missing my morning snack and getting low). Thinking back on it now, I wish there had been more flexibility.

Visiting Vancouver's Children's Hospital as a teenager was difficult. The militaristic philosophy of a strict regimen of insulin, diet and exercise, which the doctors at the hospital insisted upon, didn't leave much room to actually acknowledge that I was really just a kid. In that way I became an adult before my time, as do many children and adolescents with diabetes. Some go so far as to say that diabetes "stole" their childhood, with its demands for constant attention. As a teenager, I was expected to take on the burden immediately.

An ex-girlfriend of mine was diagnosed with diabetes as a child. I remember her saying that, as a kid, she had no idea that something was wrong. She would be in the back seat of the car in the middle of summer with the window rolled down and she'd be drooling and dreaming of the sprinklers in the fields. The thirst before diagnosis is beyond human—it's impossible to quench: you drink the water, but you're still thirsty. Your body is trying to get rid of the excess sugar in the bloodstream, so naturally that water passes through your body and you have to make many visits to the bathroom. It's not the most pleasant feeling.

Despite the difficulties involved in living with diabetes as a teenager, I was able to do most of the things my peers were doing at the time. I learned how to drive, I went to parties, I went on dates, I hung out, but I had a secret that made me different from everybody else. Ironically, I believe this has helped me come to terms with existence. If I had pretended, as the doctors and nonprofits pretend, that I could lead a "normal" life, I would be living in denial.

I was happy to graduate and to move on to the next stage in my life, which was going to Simon Fraser University to study English and Communications and working part-time. I remember Nirvana's song "Smells Like Teen Spirit" as an anthem of my 1990 graduating class, albeit from a more Americanized perspective. The lyrics resonated with the anger, horror and tension of my generation, and fit in well with the rage I felt at having diabetes. Kurt Cobain had composed his own anthem for doomed youth, but I thought it was apropos considering my own rage was boiling inside. I remember hearing the Tori Amos version and almost crying because her restrained tension and melodic piano brought it all out again.

Recently, my ten-year reunion came and went, and I resisted the urge to attend. I have not returned to my high school because it is a place that holds unhappy memories. I needed to focus on the present and not revisit the past that I had to endure. I was more than happy to leave Langley.

Building Bad Karma: Lobster Man

A hard year for me was 1993. I started full-time work in February—before that I'd only had part-time jobs while going to school. The idea was that I'd take some time off school so I'd be able to earn a degree and not be too severely mired in student loan debts.

Ironically, I realized that I was working paycheque-to-paycheque and wouldn't be any more ahead as a result of working full-time, because the pay was so meagre I couldn't save any money. I abhorred the job from the start, though I realized it was temporary, some sort of transitional period that took me to the depths, and I suffered for it.

In February, I was hired at Lobster Man. Imagine a place where the stench of seafood never leaves your clothes. Imagine coming to work in the morning and looking forward to cleaning a concrete floor and scrubbing seawater tanks of scum at the end of the day, because it means you'll be able to leave. Imagine the only respite being lunchtime, when you'd get to visit Granville Island and sit on the pier watching the seagulls dive into the water and the swarming tourists congregate around the circus where you work.

Lobster Man was a place that trapped not only crustaceans, but people. My fellow inmates included Neil, with his marine biology degree, forever commenting on certain customers' masculine good looks, much to Amaebi's disapproval. Amaebi was single and felt he had to prove his heterosexuality by helping all the women customers.

Lobster Man opened sickeningly early every morning, and that was a good thing if you were a morning person, which some regular customers were. I was no morning person. I would shave, put on jeans, a T-shirt and a fleece jacket, and hop on the Skytrain to get to work.

Once there, I'd get my boots on, tie on my apron, put on my rubber gloves and join the procession of cleaning, scrubbing and searching for dead bodies after I'd punched in on the time clock.

Butchering shellfish was a requisite task carried out by the retail staff. I remember killing my first crab.

"This is what you do," Amaebi said as the crab's legs frantically felt for footing on his rubber-gloved hands. Amaebi was clearly getting off on this, as I gasped in horror.

"Grab the crab, like this, with your fingers holding the legs and claws. Carefully."

If only the hard-shelled, writhing being in his hands could have spoken and defended itself. Amaebi brought the live crab to the sink, which had a metal piece separating the two sink basins.

"Put them on this divider, like this and crack them."

As he said it, the crab came down on the divider and was cloven in two. The bisected crab writhed, bubbles frothing from its two mouth pieces, its guts spilled into the sink. But there was little time to think about what had just happened.

I felt ill as Amaebi's gloved hands brushed crab innards into the garbage, keeping the precious white meat. He gutted the crab, cleaning out its body cavity, and dropped the pieces into the massive boiling pot.

"Now you try."

At first, it would bother anyone, but I was soon killing crabs with the rest of them. I built up a lot of negative karma at Lobster Man. It made me sick to my stomach to be subjected to killing innocent creatures for the sake of our food supply.

Despite the seafood smell, under fisheries regulations the shop had to be immaculately clean. We would scrub the concrete floor and scrub the tanks inside and out daily to keep things sterile. Garbage was stored in the freezer to keep it from stinking in the dumpster because of the summer heat.

Lobster Man involved heavy physical labour. After over a year of stable employment, and even a raise for my good work, one day I had a low blood sugar reaction on the job. I dealt with the reaction by myself, heading to the lunchroom and stuffing my face with sugar. Because nobody was allowed to leave the floor at any time, I was later called into the boss' office to explain my little drama. I told him the truth, much to my chagrin.

After he knew I had diabetes, I was somehow tarnished in

his eyes. He thought of me differently and treated me as an insurance risk—just what I wanted to avoid. He decided, ludicrously, that I was not to climb the top rungs of a ladder, which was a necessary part of the workday. Of course, the odds of my having a low blood sugar and tumbling from the top rungs were slim. He also suggested I get a job that was less strenuous physically, which seriously insulted me. Diabetes had never compromised my employment. I'd worked hard, got a raise and then, inexplicably, I was fired from Lobster Man on October 27, 1993.

They first said they fired me because of my attendance record. When they realized that my attendance was excellent and I'd even received a raise for the good work I was doing killing crustaceans full time, they said it was my poor work performance. I took them to Employment Standards for severance pay because they didn't give me two weeks notice, and ended up with a week's pay.

"You told him you had diabetes?" asked Neil.

"Yeah, I had to come out with it. He knows my medical history now. Because of that he fired me."

"But isn't that discrimination? You always pull your weight around here. You've always been great with the customers."

"Yeah, thanks. He told me not to climb up to the top tanks. As if I'd fall or something."

People with diabetes, for the most part, can tell when they are having a low blood sugar reaction. In my one and a half years with this employer, that was the only incident—an incident I dealt with alone and effectively. The reason I tell this story is to illustrate the misunderstandings some employers have about diabetes and the social stigma the condition can bring. I know that if I had told him before I was hired and put myself on the line, he would not have hired me. Now that I think back on it, maybe that would have been a good thing.

Employers often discriminate against those with diabetes. This is particularly true in the United States because employers are hesitant to cover a chronic illness when medical insurance is so expensive.

Most employers who discriminate in hiring people with diabetes cite absence as their primary concern. In fact, people with diabetes do not exceed the "normal" employee's sick days. I would even argue that managing a chronic condition oneself and keeping stable prepares one more adequately for the rigours and stress of employment.

Research has proven that the employee with diabetes is as talented and competent as one without, perhaps even more so considering the day-to-day reality of juggling diabetes. The obstacles of discrimination and licensing are frequently overcome with an almost superhuman determination to prove, beyond physical boundaries, that people with diabetes are desirable employees.

People with diabetes also frequently encounter difficulty obtaining health, life and automobile insurance, and are not eligible for military service, or scuba diving and public transport licenses.

Discrimination is unacceptable. It takes great courage and dedication to manage diabetes, and confronting ignorance of this magnitude makes it that much more difficult to manage. Employers especially have an obligation to foster a non-discriminatory atmosphere and should not see people with diabetes as disqualified on the basis of their condition.

Being honest and up front with the boss might demonstrate your maturity—or reveal the lack thereof in the boss.

Burning the Candle at Both Ends

The time I spent at Douglas College in New Westminster, and Simon Fraser University in Burnaby, and working—not to mention living—in Langley was rough, but I realized that I wanted to have a university education. I might have gone for basketball scholarships at SFU, but sports were not my focus. I wanted to focus on academics, particularly English.

Diabetes did not affect my college or university life. It was just something I dealt with on the sidelines. I spent hours sweating on the top floor of the SFU library photocopying and researching, but I ate on time, took my blood sugar and gave myself insulin injections diligently.

Today I skate, ski, swim and play guitar. I am an author. I attend a diabetes support group. I've done many things refusing to let diabetes get the better of me. It's a struggle, but I've learned to adapt.

Part Two
HIGHS AND LOWS

Chapter Four
The Diabetes Experience

The Funky Chicken

Initiation into the intricate experiences of people with diabetes includes becoming familiar with thrills such as the "funky chicken," more commonly referred to as an insulin reaction, insulin shock, low blood sugar, or in the medical textbook, "hypoglycemia." The term "funky chicken" comes from the potential convulsions that could result if the blood sugar goes too low—something that, thankfully, hasn't happened to me yet. Friends of mine with diabetes aren't as lucky.

I have heard horror stories about someone going hypo, about becoming paralyzed in jail after being picked up by the police following a night of fraternity drinking, or hearing thumping sounds only to find someone convulsing and hitting her head on the wall, or blacking out while driving and causing car accidents, or driving on the wrong side of the highway in the middle of the night. All attributed to low blood sugars. It should be noted that these are freak exceptions and not the norm; however, the experience of going hypo varies widely among people with diabetes.

Some of the symptoms that are usually associated with low blood sugar (that is, if there are any—some people don't manifest any symptoms before blacking out) are:

• Tingling of lips and tongue
• Sweating

- Nervousness
- Slurred speech
- Tremors
- Excessive hunger
- Headache
- Impaired vision
- Double vision
- Drowsiness
- Personality changes
- Confusion
- Unreasonable behaviour

This list is by no means exhaustive and has been compiled from my experience and through speaking with others who have diabetes.

People tell me I act like I'm drunk when I'm low, and judging by the symptoms, it's not that surprising. Hypoglycemia's an ugly word and an ugly experience. Any person who has diabetes knows the feeling.

I feel it in my stomach; it's a frantic, weak feeling. Sometimes I sweat, go pale and my lips tingle. I bite my lip and become irritable for no apparent reason. Later, I become panicky and I want food like there's no stopping me. It's not too pleasant having a lower than normal amount of sugar in your bloodstream. If this condition is allowed to persist, it could lead to convulsions and finally unconsciousness.

What is strange about low blood sugar is that all somebody needs to treat it is a source of sugar, such as juice, pop, candy or sugar straight up. A potentially lethal incident is cured by something as simple as sugar. If a person is unconscious, however, eating might be a problem. At this point it's either an IV with sugar and water or an injection of glucagon, the pancreatic hormone that releases glycogen from the liver.

It's a good investment to buy candy to save it for unfortunate reactions. But please don't buy that "oral gel" or those "glucose tablets," which are ridiculously expensive and prey on the diabetes market. A quick dose of sugar can be found in raisins, fruit leather, apple juice, pop, and honey, for example, which I eat to treat low blood sugar.

Of course, I'm not perfect—I've had reactions in class, at work, on trains, while sleeping, in restaurants, on the street and a variety of other places, because they're a fact of life for people who have diabetes. Luckily, I know how to recognize the symptoms and act on them before it's too late.

Going low is reality for someone with diabetes, but it can be especially traumatic to others who are around when it happens. This is a good reason to tell close friends and family that you have diabetes, so they know what to do if you go low. If you have a sugar supply on you, it's less likely to be a big problem.

How low can you go? I've actually functioned at 1.5 millimoles per litre and was able to grab a juice from the fridge at night in that state. That's a severely low blood sugar, but I've heard of worse.

So if you see your friend acting a bit drunk or irritable, it could be because she's drunk, or maybe she's just stressed from her job that day. Or she might be having an insulin reaction, in which case you should feed her something with sugar in it.

An Academy Awards show years ago had Steve Martin preparing to make a speech. I think it's an excellent example of attempted communication that goes all wrong; the kind of feeling you might have when trying to tell someone you're having an insulin reaction.

Steve Martin struts out to the podium, whooping for joy, with good intentions and audience applause. It's all fine until the audience realizes that Martin can't stop whooping—he tries to stop, but more whooping comes out of his mouth.

While Martin whoops helplessly in the background as the audience is laughing, a person approaches the podium to apologize, saying Martin is nervous and overexcited but truly wanted to introduce the next segment. It's a temporary condition. The whooping lessens in intensity, and at the very last moment before cutting to commercial, Martin finally says, "I'm okay now."

That's how it feels after going hypo: *I'm okay now. Please disregard all the previous whooping and displays of embarrassing behaviour. I've already had sugar or something to eat and it's only a matter of time before I'm back to normal. Hey, I'm okay now.*

Waiting Game

I used to have recurring dreams about saving the world. I dreamed of natural disasters, which in my sleep would act as symbolic stand-ins for my diabetes. I would find myself, for example, running with crowds of people up a hill to get away from approaching floods, all the while knowing I somehow had the ability to do something to stop the flood. Can one person make a difference in the tide of a natural disaster? Can one person rise up and conquer diabetes? In the dream, death washed over me, though life would begin again as I awoke from the panic. I would wake up sweating, unsure if I was still left in this dream of the end of the world or not.

I would test my blood sugar coming out of such dreams and find myself low. I have not had many reactions at night, but it has to be one of the worst feelings—I am left exhausted and my mind overcompensates by filling up with strange dreams.

Sometimes when eating to treat a low blood sugar, I overcompensate with food because my mind is still chanting "eat now," while my body digests what has already been eaten. It takes about 20 minutes for blood sugar levels to adjust, which is an eternity when you're low and panicky. I remember hearing about the time it takes for humans to feel full (about 20 minutes)—they don't stop eating when their stomach has filled up because their mind hasn't stopped telling them to eat. With diabetes, the mind races ahead, urging its owner to keep eating until the mind can recognize that the blood sugar is back up. That said, there is a rebound effect with low blood sugars, even if you don't overcompensate. The glucagon (a hormone produced by the pancreas that increases blood sugar in the event of low blood sugar) pushes the blood sugar up too high.

Some friends from out of town visited last year, and we hadn't seen them for a long time, so we decided to go out to a popular pasta house. I had just taken my insulin, presuming we were going to eat almost immediately after we arrived at the restaurant, so I left it at home; I'd rather not have to carry around the two bottles and a syringe if I don't have to.

You know how it is, though. You're out with friends, you talk, events and experiences are shared, and time passes quickly. Before you know it, hours have disappeared.

The line up in front of the restaurant wasn't too bad, so that was fine. But when we were seated, I knew I had a low blood sugar. I'd been enjoying the conversations up until that point, when a sudden sinking feeling set in, and I realized that over an hour had passed since my injection of lispro insulin—my low blood sugar was in full effect and we hadn't even ordered yet.

We continued talking, and suddenly the time didn't disappear so quickly anymore. It seemed to drag because I was now conscious of my low blood sugar. My mind raced thinking of possible outlets—perhaps some pop. Ordering a drink would take too long. I needed to weigh the options and do something quickly. Because the restaurant was so busy, we weren't getting our meal any time soon.

It would have been nice to have had something in my pocket for an unfortunate moment such as this, but I had nothing.

Then I saw packets of sugar on the table. I smiled at everyone, took two packages of sugar, and proceeded to pour them into my hand.

"I have diabetes," I explained to my wide-eyed companions, and that's all I could explain in that state. I wolfed the sugar into my mouth.

These are the moments that feed the rumour mill of diabetes. *He was eating sugar,* they might say. *People with diabetes aren't supposed to eat sugar. How strange. He must have been cheating on his diet.* With friends, it's one thing. With business partners or in a foreign country, I can imagine how people might react to such a display. But who cares what other people think? Would they rather have someone lying on the floor waiting for an ambulance?

Despite my thoughts about the rumour mill, one of my friends proceeded to take some sugar packets for himself, remarking how good they tasted.

"Yummy! I could get used to this," he exclaimed as he dumped the sugar into his hand and poured it into his mouth.

"What?" he said, as I looked at him in disbelief. "I'm starving too, you know."

On Top of the World

There's nothing like standing on top of a mountain. You seem to be on top of the world, looking down into valleys of green cedar trees and snow-capped peaks.

I took a ski trip up to Whistler, B.C., a world-renowned ski resort. The expense of a lift ticket is considerable, so it's not often that I have the privilege to put two planks on my feet and make my way down groomed slopes of snow. I was bundled up in layers of clothing to fight off the cold and was all geared up with skis, poles and goggles.

I took the quad chair up higher and higher, hearing the swish of snowboarders and skiers making their way down the mountain, cutting and carving the slopes. The lift cables rocked back and forth in the biting wind.

I pushed off the lift platform once I reached the top, steadying myself as I left the safety of the lift, and found myself standing on top of the world. I remember the ice crystals falling magically from my mouth as my breath froze, and the chill wind that carried them along the snow's surface, which was smooth and coated with an icy dust. It's strange to look down on other mountains, realizing you're actually higher than them, seeing pristine snow on their tips, the reflection of sun off their polar caps, and trees descending into the valley. Perhaps this is the delirium of height.

I like skiing. There's a peace about it. I'm not into extreme skiing and haven't tried snowboarding yet, but I might someday. But skiing posed a special problem after I'd prepared to battle the cold and eaten a big breakfast. I had taken the lift up and skied down many times before I suddenly realized I had lost my ability to ski.

What was most strange about wiping out and biting snow is that I blamed it on my skiing ability. I'm not a professional—definitely intermediate—so there were no black diamonds for me. But this particular section was giving me trouble. I would get back up, only to fall again miserably while others skied around me. One guy even stopped to ask if I was all right—of course I was all right. I got back up again and did the most spectacular wipe out I'd done in a while, losing one ski and almost dislocating my leg and arm in the process. Everything was fine, I thought, until I realized I was low.

That explained it. That was what I had forgotten. For a blissful half day, I had actually forgotten about diabetes—and what bliss. But now I was low and needed something to eat to bring my blood sugar back up to normal in a hurry. I hadn't eaten enough food, because insulin absorbs faster in an active body. Luckily, I had packed some fruit leather for just such an occasion, so I wasn't too troubled. But it was there, sitting on a snowy slope with skiers and snowboarders flying past me, that I realized that diabetes was something I'd always have to think about, no matter what I did.

After I'd consumed sugar, I was fine. With rubbery legs I got up and skied the rest of the day, breaking for lunch and realizing by trial and error that skiing took a lot of energy and extra food to enjoy, or a reduction in insulin. Diabetes has not stopped me from skiing.

Getting High

Understandably, some people like getting high. When someone with diabetes is talking about getting high, however, it's not so fun. Having blood go extra sweet is called hyperglycemia in the textbook. There's nothing hyper about it, except that your blood fills up with extra sugar. Symptoms for the other end of the blood sugar spectrum include:

- Excessive thirst
- Excessive urination
- Nausea
- Vomiting
- Drowsiness
- Acetone breath
- Flushed skin

These symptoms are often similar to the ones experienced with the initial onset of diabetes. Excessive thirst is what tells me I'm high, not to mention nausea. Fortunately, I seldom get to the vomiting stage.

If left too long in the hyperglycemic condition, a person with diabetes can lapse into a coma and can even die; as with low blood sugar, however, the symptoms can often be recognized and treated. High blood sugar is dealt with by injecting insulin. Ketoacidosis is a condition that is brought on if the blood sugar has been high too long and the body starts trying to burn fat for fuel, producing acid (ketones) that build up in the body, spilling into the urine. This may happen if an insulin dose is missed or an infection occurs, for instance.

Essentially, then, the goal is to avoid getting both low and high and maintain the idyllic blood sugar between 4 and 8 millimoles per litre. Nonetheless, highs and lows happen, and it's part of diabetes. I find after a low blood sugar, my body overcompensates (or I eat too much to get back to a stable blood sugar). With experience it becomes easier to determine how your body works and how much you need to eat to level out.

All this being said, Suzanne Bennett Johnson of the University of Florida Health Sciences Centre writes:

Although the goal of treatment is to maintain the patient's blood glucose levels within the normal range, current methods of exogenous insulin replacement (that's what you're doing when you inject insulin) only crudely approximate normal pancreatic function. Consequently, both "hyperglycemia" (excessively high blood sugar) and "hypoglycemia" (excessively low blood sugar, also known as "insulin shock") can and do occur. [11]

Indeed, insulin can only "crudely approximate normal pancreatic function." Insulin can only control a blood sugar if it is used alongside myriad other lifestyle changes. Nobody's perfect. Doctors cannot expect patients to be perfect. Doing your best is all anyone can ask.

Chapter 5
The Diabetes Front Line

Burden of Responsibility

Diabetes demands a certain do-it-yourself (DIY) approach to treatment, which places much of the responsibility for care in the hands of the affected person. I was discharged from the hospital just over one week after I was diagnosed, and since then it's been injections, blood tests and a strictly regimented diet. This sort of DIY treatment is difficult because the burden is squarely on the shoulders of the person with diabetes. In terms of the day-to-day aspects of diabetes management, the responsibility shifts from the medical system to the affected person.

The DIY approach to diabetes care is not something that is chosen. There is simply nobody but yourself to actually administer the insulin and test your blood sugar. It requires a daily consideration of dosages, how your body will react to certain foods and how exercise and your job will affect blood sugar levels, among other things.

This has its beneficial aspects, such as the ability to dose insulin depending on the results of blood sugar monitoring, to eat a variety of foods and to participate in exercise activities. But it can also backfire if a physician equates an individual's treatment choices with moral decisions or blames a patient for not "complying" with a prescribed regimen.

The fact is that high blood sugars or a high Hemoglobin A1c result do not necessarily mean that the person with diabetes has not attempted to follow a particular regimen, even though a physician may blame the patient for exactly that. There are many factors that affect blood sugar levels. Hormones and stress, for example, may increase or decrease blood sugar, depending upon the individual. Blaming the patient is particularly damaging in the context of a DIY treatment, especially when assumptions are made about a condition that is still misunderstood, misdiagnosed and not easily predictable.

Physicians should not blame people with diabetes for developing complications. It may be that such complications relate to lifestyle choices, but it is also true that everybody reacts differently. One person might follow a physician's advice religiously and develop complications anyway. Another might only follow a physician's advice when it suits him or her but still not develop any complications at all. Complications can develop because of lifestyle choices, but they might also arise from genetic factors, which cannot be predicted.

We understand that a healthy body is a suitable goal most of the time, but there is an assumption that "perfect" health is the natural state of a human being. This is a common assumption in holistic medicine. By contrast, conventional medicine treats diseases, not people. Human beings, however, have all kinds of things going on in their bodies about which they have no clue, and neither kind of medicine can supply all the answers.

Ultimately, it is the person with diabetes who shoulders the responsibility for directing his or her treatment. Physicians, dieticians or other medical professionals may offer advice based on their education and experience, but a person with diabetes often lears by trial and error what works and what doesn't for his or her own body. Certainly an endocrinologist may recognize trends in blood sugar levels and suggest solutions such as insulin adjustments, but practical solutions are often arrived at through experience. For example, I learned much more about diabetes from attending a diabetes support group than I did attending all my appointments with my family physician in the years prior to 1994. What I learned about the day-to-day reality of diabetes in the experiential environment, as opposed to the conventional medical one, was invaluable.

I must have stabbed myself over a thousand times—you begin to feel like a pincushion with all the finger pokes to test blood, not to mention the insulin injections.

I take two different types of insulin—regular (short acting) and NPH (long acting) human insulin. I am currently changing the regular insulin to lispro insulin (extra-short acting). Some people with diabetes still take animal-based insulin, derived from cows or pigs (known as beef insulin and pork insulin), but pharmaceutical companies decided to phase it out because of a yet unexplained reason likely attributed market forces. Unfortunately, because both insulin types seem to affect the body differently, some people with diabetes who were used to animal insulin and subsequently switched to human insulin, couldn't tell when they were getting low. In the worst cases, this led to death.

Regular insulin starts lowering my blood sugar about a half hour after injection and peaks about 2 to 4 hours after the dose, for an overall effect lasting about 6 to 8 hours. For a while I used lispro insulin, because it reacts more quickly, beginning to work only 5 to 15 minutes after injection, peaking in an hour, and leaving my system in, at most, 4 hours.

Just after I began my treatment with lispro insulin I found it was not covered under my medical plan, therefore I pay full price. Despite being prescribed lispro insulin, I have reverted to regular insulin because of the expense. (This is one of the problems with the health care system in Canada, which is beginning to model itself on the privatized healthcare of the U.S. If I moved to the U.K. right now, I would be covered for everything. As it is I have to pay an expensive deductible, and even after I pay that, I only get 80 percent back. But I count my blessings that I haven't had to pay the full cost of treatment, which would be crippling at this stage.)

NPH insulin starts lowering my blood sugar about 1 to 3 hours after injection and peaks about 6 to 12 hours after the dose. The overall effect lasts about 18 to 24 hours.

Waking up in the morning can be a bit of a problem. I find if my blood sugar is high, it's harder to get up. Lethargy is not the most appealing aspect of a high blood sugar. Things can be done to correct the problem, though, such as adjusting insulin dosages or going to bed earlier. Insomnia is a problem, although in my case, it probably has more to do with the invention of the electric light bulb and television than diabetes.

If I wake up and my blood sugar is around the ideal range of four to eight, I feel great. I wake up refreshed and ready to start the day. Shortly after I wake up, I take a shot of insulin. I store my supply in the fridge—except the bottles I'm currently using, one each of regular insulin (or lispro insulin) and NPH insulin. Out of the fridge, insulin is

Good Health Eating Guide Choices

The following categoriesmake up *The Good Health Eating Guide*. Each example of food makes up one category choice (i.e., one starch would be one slice of bread):

1. Starch (15 grams carbohydrate):
• 1 slice of bread
• 1/2 cup of cereal
• 2 cookies
• 1/2 a potato
• 1/2 cup of pasta

2. Fruit and vegetable (10 grams carbohydrate):
• 1/2 an apple
• 1 orange
• 1 cup watermelon
• 1/2 cup of carrots

3. Milk (6 grams carbohydrate):
• 1/2 cup of milk
• 1/2 cup of plain yogurt

4. Sugar (10 grams carbohydrate):
• 2 hard candies
• 2 marshmallows
• 1/2 cup regular pop

5. Protein:
- 1 chicken leg
- 1 ounce of fish
- 1 egg

6. Fats and oils:
- 1 teaspoon mayonnaise
- 1 slice of bacon
- 1 teaspoon butter

7. Extra:
- Lettuce
- Bean sprouts
- Broccoli
- Asparagus

supposed to last a month.

Rotating injection sites is a good idea, so as not to build up scar tissue in one area. I seldom break the syringe after using it, because it's still usable a few more times, after which it becomes dull and is painful to inject. I don't like the idea of these syringes taking up space a landfill site, so I recycle by using the syringe as many times as I can. This is especially useful when travelling, although it is not recommended by health professionals.

Insulin is injected just below the skin, in the layer of fat—this is called "subcutaneous injection." This is so it can be absorbed effectively to approximate a consistent blood sugar. Insulin is not, despite what many people think, injected into a vein.

Sometimes when you inject insulin, you hit a blood vessel that bleeds and can make a nasty bruise at the injection site. Fortunately, this doesn't happen often. I give myself insulin in my stomach, legs, thigh, lower back or butt. I don't like injecting into my arms because it's awkward and I would hit my muscle, which would be painful and the insulin would absorb too quickly.

Yes, injecting insulin can be painful. No, it's not exactly fun. But some injections are more painful than others. It becomes routine, a daily drama required to survive.

The nurses told me I'd get used to it. They said it would be like brushing my teeth. It's not. A better analogy might be taking shock therapy to improve your mental health. Or maybe something less extreme, such as taking a pill. Insulin cannot, unfortunately, be taken orally.

I remember reading somewhere that the part of the pancreas that produces insulin is about as big as the tip of your smallest finger. How could something so small have such a huge physiological effect? How could some tiny part of this important digestive organ—the pancreas—be responsible for so much?

If you add up the years people with diabetes spend treating it and the possible complications that may result, it becomes clear that diabetes isn't just some minor bug that's been cured. It demands attention even at the most inopportune times and can get serious very rapidly.

Assuming I test my blood sugar, which I do almost every morning, and take my insulin, I can get up and take on the world. Immediately after breakfast, that is, because it's only a matter of time before the blood sugar starts to lower, an effect that can only be counteracted with sugar, which means food. (In an extreme case, such as when travelling, I have found I can cut out my regular insulin altogether and not eat breakfast, but I wouldn't endorse that because you tend to get hungry.)

Breakfast usually includes all the food groups, but I no longer have any scales and do not weigh my food or measure exactly, like I used to in the early days when my parents and I were learning.

The Good Health Eating Guide was devised by a group of dieticians at the Canadian Diabetes Association (CDA) to simplify the diabetes diet. Suspiciously similar to *Canada's Food Guide to Healthy Living*—and with almost the same name—it recommended a bland diet from the four major food groups.

I followed this diet religiously in the beginning, narrowing all foods down into six categories: starch, fruit and vegetable, milk, protein, fats and oils, and extra choices.

Sugar at the time was completely avoided (there used to be no sugar choice at all) and that is why the general public today still thinks that people with diabetes cannot eat sugar. In 1994, the CDA decided to add sugar choices, which could be interchanged with fruits and vegetables. For example, one popsicle equaled 10 grams of carbohydrates, roughly the equivalent of a small orange or half a pear. Suffice it to say that such a regimen made eating an extremely unpleasant ordeal and necessitated a meat-and-potatoes existence. Of course, I could always find consolation in the "extra" food choices, by pigging out on unlimited asparagus or broccoli, or by scarfing a few heads of lettuce and a few cucumbers. It makes the mouth water.

I have learned by experience, however, to figure out in my head how various food groups will react. Sometimes, I admit, I get it wrong, but experience is a good teacher. I don't usually make the same mistake twice.

Adjusting insulin and food is a fine art. Yes, it's true that one should eat from all food groups, but carbohydrate content is much different in beans than in tuna. All food eventually breaks down into sugar and fat, with simple sugars the quickest to push up a blood sugar and fats the slowest. I try to focus on the carbohydrate content, because it's a more accurate measure of what I'm eating.

When I was riding my bike to work I had to compensate by eating more food for breakfast and lowering my insulin intake in the morning. I always brought juice in case I got low mid-route, but that hardly ever happened. It's not ideal to work out on a full stomach, but what can you do? Biking to and from work rounded out the desk job nicely. (In fact, my employer had no clue that I had diabetes, though I worked there over a full year before travelling to Europe.)

At lunchtime, I seldom test my blood sugar, but have a light snack. Dinnertime means another insulin shot. The shot at dinner is usually adjusted to my blood sugar result, as is the morning dosage. If I am out at a restaurant, I bring a syringe and both the NPH and regular insulin with me in a plastic freezer bag. The blood test machine is still too cumbersome for me to carry around—you have to give those pincushion fingers a rest sometime.

Another option for taking insulin is a pump that attaches to your body and delivers regular doses of insulin. It allows for greater mobility, but there are drawbacks. I have chosen not to use a pump for financial concerns more than anything else. The pump costs thousands of dollars. Two types of insulin and a syringe cost about $60. Also, you still have to rotate injection sites, as you would if you were using needles, and the pump is attached to you at all times. I've decided the pump isn't for me right now, but some people find it's a great alternative to traditional injections.

I have a friend who will never stop using the pump. For him, it's become something more than just a machine—it's bound up in a concept of freedom and choice. He now has the ability to decide on the fly to go out with co-workers to a restaurant after work. With insulin, he might have had to go home and shoot up first. It also supplies a constant dosage of insulin, instead of a large dose all at once. The down side is that if the pump shut off, ran out of insulin or malfunctioned, then it would be a matter of hours before ketoacidosis set in. The traditional bottles of insulin and a syringe are kept on hand at home just in case.

Many athletes have taken to the pump because it's the latest, greatest, most accurate way to manage diabetes. I am not a professional athlete, but if it works for them or for you, that's great. Right now, I can barely afford the Pharmacare deductible each year, let alone thousands for an insulin pump.

Testing my blood sugar involves pricking my finger with a lancet-loaded poking device. It reminds me sometimes of the bloodletting that was done to treat patients in the past. In the past, physicians attempted to cure people of their illnesses by actually letting someone bleed to cleanse them of their sickness.

Not surprisingly, many people died because of blood loss, not because of their illness. Every day blood tests force me to see blood on my fingertips before each meal, as if I was somehow curing myself through bloodletting or conducting amateur chemistry experiments.

Ironically, I remember sitting in biology class before my diagnosis, when I was about fourteen years old. The biology teacher wanted us to prick our fingers to see what blood type each of us was. Everyone in the class found out their blood types, but not me; I had an unnatural aversion to having my finger poked with a sharp object even before I had diabetes.

As with injection sites, finger pokes have to be rotated. I squeeze a bead of blood out of my finger, which is more difficult if the finger is cold or if the lancet is dull. Yes, it is painful. No it's not like brushing your teeth. More like flagellating yourself over some religious icon. If the blood sugar reading is low, I drink juice or consume another sugar product to bring it up.

The only sure way to know if you're low or high is testing your blood sugar; you'll be able to adjust your insulin accordingly by recognizing trends (average readings) over time.

The only time I was extremely low was while travelling in Europe. I was in St. Albans and had just been to London on the train. I was with my wife and daughter.

I knew I was low when I got off the train and had already stuffed my face with candies. Unfortunately, it wasn't enough—or was too little too late. I remember walking up the street and becoming tired, and again my mind was racing, so I thought I should sit down. I believe I did sit down, but at some point I got back up and fell on the sidewalk with my legs out in the road—not exactly an ideal position to be in. It was a Saturday night, and I remember thinking that the passers-by must all assume that I was drunk.

It was a waiter from the Café des Amis in St. Albans who responded to my wife's search for help. It's almost impossible to believe that a simple glass of juice saved me from a visit to the hospital. I put my wife and daughter through a scare, after which I came back to consciousness as if nothing had happened. Relying on others for help is all right.

As for the other end of the blood sugar spectrum, the highest I've been was when I was diagnosed at 42 millimoles per litre. I was lucky that I did not slip into a hyperglycemic coma.

Dinner means more food that I don't weigh on a scale—I know that a glass of milk covers the milk choices or that a cup of yogurt does the same. The variety of a diet cannot be emphasized enough—variety is what makes life interesting. I have to admit that occasionally I fall into the fast food syndrome of our culture and eat prepared meals, but nothing can beat real food. You know, food that's actually cooked and has more complexity than an opened can of beans.

The recommended diet for people with diabetes has become looser in recent years. Starvation diets are no longer in vogue, as they were in the times before insulin. Sugars are now a meal choice. I still try to have fruit and vegetables, which have more natural forms of sugar, like fructose. It is, however, nice to know that I can have ice cream once in a while.

I usually have a small snack before bed. I might also test at this time to make sure I'm on track. I don't like eating anything before bed, but if I don't, I'll get low at night. I always, thankfully, wake up when I fall too low while sleeping. I know as soon as I wake up that I need to eat. I'm hungry, thirsty and I usually sweat. (Thirst is a strange instinct when it comes to diabetes. It's never possible to be absolutely sure what the thirst means. I'm thirsty when I'm high and thirsty when I'm low. Other times, I'm just thirsty. It's hard to tell sometimes whether I'm thirsty because of diabetes, or merely because I'm dehydrated.)

Being low at night makes me overcompensate. Because of the extreme hunger, I eat. With increased nighttime eating, there is weight gain, as all the extra sugar in the bloodstream is stored as fat while you sleep.

That being said, those with diabetes are not all overweight.

Obesity is, however, a contributing factor to type 2 diabetes, so there is much confusion as to the average person with diabetes' stature. People with diabetes should also keep an eye on their weight, but so should those without diabetes. Talking with a doctor and dietician can help those with diabetes determine a manageable weight loss or gain plan.

Curse of the Chocolate Covered Almonds

One day I ate some chocolate covered almonds, which I'll admit is not exactly the healthiest diet for anybody, let alone someone with diabetes. I compensated for this intake of extraneous food by taking lispro insulin, therefore counteracting the ensuing rise in blood sugar.

Before you jump to conclusions about my diabetes control, note that my blood sugar did not travel above the ideal boundaries of a normal blood sugar range. Don't worry. I compensated.

Does my eating those chocolate almonds mean I should feel guilty? Should I flagellate myself or pray? Might I be bestowing myself with bad karma associated with almonds? Should I be concerned about the addictive properties of chocolate?

This is the way a person with diabetes may have to think sometimes. Weighing the options and making choices about what one is consuming, then living with the consequences, is what living with diabetes is all about. Do I consider myself a cheater? No. Will I be rewarded if I abstain from certain foods I enjoy because they might negatively affect me? No.

The argument might be framed better if the whole world was told diligently by physicians and pharmaceutical companies that many research trials and scientific studies had shown that chocolate almonds were just plain bad for you. And maybe they could give out medals to people who abstained from sex for that matter; because of course, the desire for sex and food are two of the most powerful and basic instincts in human beings. Enforcing celibacy is quite similar to enforcing a strict diet in many respects.

I bought the almonds from a thirteen-year-old boy who was

selling boxes at three dollars a pop for a group that, according to the back of the box, imparts "valuable business experience, confidence, and a sense of responsibility and leadership." How could I refuse?

I suppose it's time to confess all. I remember having some icing on a cookie, too. Does that count as cheating? Shall I be chastised? Getting through any given holiday is a feat in itself. Around Christmas, forgive me, I consumed—it grieves me to say it—potato chips and even a beer. (I remember reading an article in a magazine saying that beer is actually good for you, or was that a glass of wine?)

Is nothing sacred anymore? I can hear them now in the streets shouting for me. Come out with your hands up. Maybe they could put all those who sell chocolate almonds in jail. Arrest the whole lot of them, and candy manufacturers too, for that matter. Maybe it'd be like a modern day chocolate almond prohibition, where people would surreptitiously sneak to night-clubs and hide the almonds inside potato chip bags, just like they tried to hide alcohol in pop bottles during prohibition. People would be picked up on the street for overdosing on chocolate almonds and lying in the gutter. You might relate this dietary nightmare to something you've eaten or craved one day.

One day I craved sushi. We went to a restaurant just down the street for its handmade sushi; probably the best I'd ever tasted. They made it right there in front of you. Here's a question to perplex all you dieticians out there. What is sushi? How to deal with a meal of sushi? Rice, fish and seaweed should be easy enough to figure out when it comes to that insulin dosage. But what if you throw in a few dynamite rolls and maybe a gyoza or two? Not to mention a bit of ginger at the end of it all. Then you're in trouble.

What about Caesar salad? Or spring rolls? Or the sprouts in chow mein? What about samosas or papads? Indulge in some serious ethnic cooking here in multicultural Canada and we might run into some insulin dosage problems. It makes little sense that, in a diverse country such as Canada, dieticians receive pats on the back from the medical community—which has finally recognized the importance of diet for people with diabetes—for promoting the proper insulin dosages to take with potatoes and ham.

Diet is important for people with type 1 diabetes, but not nearly as important as it is for person who has spent a lifetime gaining weight by eating greasy fast food, has type 2 diabetes at age 53 and needs to take some pills. I think there's a difference here—the five-year-old child with diabetes who takes insulin doesn't need to be assessed using the same guidelines as the overweight 53 year old, because no two people are the same. Everyone has a different metabolism, and thus different insulin and medication needs.

Diet is one of the factors that lead to illness, even according to the Hippocratic oath, which is still recited by physicians today. It's not the only thing, however, to consider when diagnosing an illness.

Nuts aren't the greatest things for blood sugars. They are just about pure fat, so their effect on your body will appear much later because they're not absorbed into the metabolism as quickly as, for example, a chocolate almond. Wait a second. That's both a nut and chocolate. Sugar straight up, with a bit of fat to take effect a bit later. Maybe those chocolate almonds weren't such a good idea after all.

The fact is, just about anything can be included into a person with diabetes' diet. But that doesn't mean overeating—it means you have choices, just like anybody else in the world. People with diabetes aren't aliens. You don't have to tread lightly and be overly concerned about their feelings around food.

I don't know how many times I've been a dinner guest and my hosts have made all sorts of assumptions about what I can and cannot eat. I'm damned if I eat and I'm damned if I don't, or so it seems. I admit there are people with diabetes who need to follow certain dietary requirements, such as a low salt diet because of heart disease or abstinence from alcohol because of liver damage. This is indisputable. People need to listen to the recommendations of their doctor, but take them with a grain of salt (no pun intended).

I was just hungry, that's all.

Cigarettes, Alcohol and other Drugs

It is inevitable that some people with diabetes smoke, some are obese, some also drink more alcohol than others, and some probably drink too much coffee. Much of this comes down to individual choices.

Medical professionals take it upon themselves to warn of possible consequences of smoking, drinking and doing drugs. In the plethora of books written by doctors, dietitians and nurses, there is much information on the devastating effects of smoking, alcohol and other drugs. These books often break the issues down into moral absolutes, as do many books on diabetes.

According to these books, you must test your blood sugar. You have to quit smoking because it causes your blood vessels to constrict. You have to stay away from alcohol and illegal drugs altogether. And the best of all, you must not eat any sugar.

I plead for moderation and a non-judgemental attitude. A regimented, strict and stifling diet will not be followed. People need to want to change before they can take the steps to changing their lifestyles. Minimizing the impact of diabetes on the person with diabetes' lifestyle is imperative. Forcing a person with diabetes to make a multitude of changes all at once is simply ineffective, if not impossible.

Diabetes radically changes a person's lifestyle; there is no question about that. But it's not a medical professional's role to be a police officer, even though they often assume that role. It is the patient's responsibility to learn everything he or she can from the sources of information at their disposal: doctors, family and friends with diabetes, diabetes support groups, books on diabetes and endocrinologists.

Regardless, certain practices are unhealthy whether you have diabetes or not. Smoking, for instance, is known to introduce your lungs to a host of 4,000 chemicals and poisons such as arsenic, carbon monoxide, cyanide and formaldehyde. Forty-three of these chemicals are known cancer-causing agents (carcinogens).

Any doctor can tell you to stop smoking until they are blue in the face (and black in the lungs), but people will still smoke. My grandmother smoked and died of lung cancer. It's not something I choose to have in my life. There are too many reasons not to smoke—not the least of which being the expense of cigarettes. I know that people with diabetes will still smoke, and it is not up to me to preach. It is you who has to decide to choose what is right for you. But you should also be aware of the possible consequences of your actions, in order to make informed decisions about them.

Alcohol actually lowers the blood sugar, unless it's loaded with sugar as some alcoholic drinks are. If a doctor has a valid reason why you should not drink alcohol, then you have to weigh the advantages and the disadvantages.

I encourage any person with diabetes to experiment on how alcohol affects the blood sugar by testing it after a pint of beer. Low blood sugar is a risk when drinking—not only does alcohol lower the blood sugar, but if you suffer a reaction, people might think you're drunk and leave you collapsed in the corner, which could lead to a severe reaction and perhaps even death. This is a good reason to abstain altogether, but if you must drink, I find eating a little extra works well for me. Learn how your body reacts to alcohol and drink responsibly.

Wine is fine in moderation, of course. So are lager beers and light ales that don't have large sugar contents. Spirits, like rum, whiskey and vodka are also fine with diet pop mixers—in moderation.

Drugs pose a significant risk to one's health, even alcohol and nicotine, both of which are legalized drugs. Drugs that are illegal have more risk attached to them in the sense that they are forced underground.

The reality is that some people will choose to use drugs. Instead of trying to stop young people with diabetes from taking drugs, it makes more sense to educate them about how various recreational drugs will interact with diabetes.

It's no surprise that drug use is a risky practice, but for a person with diabetes, those risks are intensified. For example, the common and easily obtainable drug marijuana can pose significant risks for a person with diabetes. The most immediate and potentially dangerous effect is the craving for sweets and the intense hunger one may experience directly after using marijuana. Giving into this increase in appetite can lead to high blood sugar.

If a person with diabetes chooses to use illegal narcotics, or even alcohol or cigarettes, it's important that he or she take steps to minimize those risks. It's advisable to contact various diabetes associations (some of which are listed at the end of this book) if you have any questions regarding alcohol, cigarette or recreational drug use and diabetes.

Chapter 6
Coming Out of the Closet

Each person with diabetes somehow faces the realities of living with a chronic condition, whether they want to or not. Something has to happen inside to make a person actually proceed with treatment or not. What makes diabetes even more difficult, beyond the daily injections, blood tests and dietary restrictions, is discrimination.

On the outside, a person with diabetes looks perfectly normal, and it's a hard struggle to decide whether coming out of the closet with diabetes in certain situations will bring support or stigma. If people are so blatantly discriminatory when it comes to things like pilot licensing, scuba diving, giving blood and driving, it's no small wonder that people with diabetes don't volunteer the information to everyone they meet.

We might say that discrimination on the basis of religion or race is wrong; that prejudice or bias does not recognize the other as an individual. What about discrimination on the basis of a known medical condition such as diabetes? For example, a varsity coach may decide not to play a team member with diabetes because he or she may have an insulin reaction. While this fear may be justified to protect the school's liability in the event of an accident, it is a fear based on misunderstanding of diabetes.

To face diabetes is a massive challenge, especially to those who are newly diagnosed. Even those who have had it for years hit rough times, though it does get easier with time to establish a routine. As limiting as diabetes may seem, it does not have to cripple. Life is valuable despite the juggling.

The reality is that people with diabetes are discriminated against in all walks of life. Three of the most serious areas are employment, vehicle licensing (and licensing in general) and school. Constantly having to justify diabetes and explain it to others is frustrating and exhausting. Rumours are often unfounded and are based on misinformation and ignorance, but they've usually already done their damage. People with diabetes are just that—people—not an illness. They are marathon runners. They are teachers. They are doctors. They are successful in many different walks of life.

People who do not understand others may fear their differences rather than live with them. This is the basis for racism, sexism and other forms of discrimination. It is not my goal to add another "ism" to the list, but discrimination against those with diabetes exists and we must work towards accepting people. Ignorance of other people's life experiences is a condition more crippling to the world than diabetes will ever be.

People with diabetes, crucially, are not burdens to society. Employers often cite fear and apprehension that a person with diabetes presents a safety risk to the employer or the public. Such fear is often based on misinformation or a lack of up-to-date knowledge about diabetes. Many people with diabetes know when they are having a low blood sugar because there are often warning signs such as rapid heartbeat, sweating, shakiness, anxiety and hunger. People with diabetes should be evaluated on an individual basis and should not be excluded from employment on the basis of their diabetes. All people with diabetes are not the same.

Unfortunately, employers particularly discriminate against people with type 1 diabetes. This is despite the fact that when people with diabetes are hired, their "employment experiences...appear to be similar to the experiences of the nondiabetic population..." and "absenteeism among (insulin dependent diabetes) cases currently working did not differ from that of the nondiabetic siblings," according to a 1989 research study. [12]

Mind Your Labels

Criminology is the study of crime, and many theories attempt to explain why people engage in criminality. Labelling theory [13] is one perspective from criminology that has particularly interesting applications to discussions about diabetes and discrimination.

Labelling theory contends that formal labels placed on offenders influence their likelihood to continue as offenders. In other words, if I call you criminal, process you through the criminal justice system as a criminal, and charge you with offenses under the criminal code that label you, for example, as a thief, then you are stuck with that label. It's on your criminal record. It comes up wherever you go, from school to employment. You can't leave the country. The power of this societal label is extremely strong and often stigmatizes an individual to the point where they internalize the label.

Human beings respond according to the definitions that are placed upon their behaviour by others, particularly by those in power, such as court judges or physicians. Repeated acts of deviance are often the consequence of a formal label because tags such as "criminal," "delinquent" or "thief" eventually alter an individual's self-image to the point where they begin to identify themself as the label and act accordingly. [14]

Labelling theorists contend that only groups in power, usually white males, are the ones who define formal laws at the expense of those who are unable to effect change on the system. If we take the example of the criminal justice system, we see that those lacking sufficient power, such as minorities, are most likely labelled as criminals, and people who are executives in office buildings are not. This also has to do with the visibility of the crime and its enforceability.

Moreover, those who lack the necessary resources are more likely to be labelled since they cannot hire competent lawyers to successfully defend themselves. As Howard Becker puts it, "...social groups create deviance by making the rules whose infraction constitutes deviance, and by applying those rules to particular people and labelling them as outsiders." [15] These "outsiders" are pushed to the margins of society.

Labelling theorists argue that a person labelled as a criminal is more likely to continue reinforcing such behaviour, as they are not only shunned by conformist peers, but are accepted into the groups who are already labelled criminal. This results in a downward spiral as the "criminal" is forced to associate with fellow criminals, pushing them further away from people who might reinforce a more positive definition of self.

The assumptions of labelling theory have some validity; many practitioners within the criminal justice system are currently making more of an effort not to stigmatize those who may be more sensitive to labels, such as juvenile delinquents. Many treatment and prevention programs now attempt to build positive self-images instead of creating negative tags, which to some degree proves labelling theory's legitimacy.

We all to some extent internalize the labels others apply to us—especially labels applied by those in power. We even rely on stereotypical notions of who a person is by their appearance, and, as I've argued, by their connections to roles of status and scientific legitimacy. As James Wilson and Patricia Rachel have written in "Can the Government Regulate Itself?", it is a known fact that you could:

> Dress a person in a three-piece suit, let him grow a beard, and what he says will prove more believable to most audiences than the same message delivered by the same person dressed in jeans and looking casual and unimpressive. [16]

This means to say the same message coming from the mouth of a physician and coming from a person with diabetes is seen in different ways—one carries more authority and legitimacy than the other. This puts me in an awkward position, and it's more about public perceptions and assumptions about people who occupy a position of power than it is about the accuracy of the message.

Labelling theory extends beyond criminology—its ideas resurface in areas such as the health care system. The practice of medicine, like the justice system, has a habit of labelling people. If I am labelled "diabetic" and treated as a diabetic, and am not expected to be anything more than a diabetic, the labelling is detrimental. As a person, I might internalize this identity and not allow myself to break free from the constraints of this condition. It is especially debilitating when it's a chronic condition, because the person must confront it continually through checkups at the doctors, visits with the pharmacist, family members, friends and even each day through blood testing and insulin injections.

There is another set of labels people use, but they are to designate authority. They are "police officer" or "lawyer" or "doctor" or "priest." Respect is afforded to people who embody such labels—these abstract roles imply status—but they are only roles that society has imbued with power. Wouldn't labels such as these occupations serve better than the label "diabetic"? In fact, you can be a lawyer who happens to have diabetes.

Breaking away from the label "diabetic" is easier said than done. I have argued elsewhere in this book that the actual naming of the medical condition is problematic also—the terminology carries with it a legacy of science, misunderstandings and confusion. A child who takes insulin injections and a senior citizen who takes pills and adjusts his or her diet are both labelled "diabetic" as if both experience the same things following diagnosis. Diabetes covers a wide range of conditions and treatments and is not adequately dealt with by one label from the medical community. A more comprehensive approach to diabetes might be in order. Such an approach would allow people to experience life without the negative labels.

I was christened as "diabetic" by an authoritative physician at diagnosis. A whole set of stigmatizing baggage that I didn't know existed came along with the actual physical condition. While applying this label isn't considered as drastic as the process of law enforcement labelling a criminal, it has a similar negative connotation in that it brands someone as a disease, rather than recognizing the fullness of their humanity. I would rather be considered on the merits of my interests and character traits than on a physiological condition.

The label may even have the adverse effect of an individual rebelling against the condition or not seeking medical treatment from fear of reprimand from the physician who has assumed the role of a police officer. Obviously, it is not the place of a physician to make moralistic assumptions about lifestyle, especially if the assumptions come from a single Hemoglobin A1c result being "bad."

My family physician, for example, suggested my Hemoglobin A1c was "too high," though he didn't exactly say it was "bad." The result was, however, reasonable within the boundaries my diabetes specialist and I had set. I was on the right track.

With such varying reactions between physicians I realized that physicians are not always on the right track themselves. I decided to take the diabetes specialist's recommendations to heart because the family physician was just second-guessing. Be careful with what people in authority tell you and make sure it jibes with you as a person.

Needlephobia

> I suppose I am sort of a drug addict now. I am addicted to insulin, which I inject several times a day. I do not mind the injections; they have become routine, like cleaning my teeth in the morning. [17]

Even Theresa McLean has used the drug addict metaphor, which seems to be lodged in the public's psyche surrounding needles. Bad experiences with needles abound; people wince when they take injections to protect them from diseases. The syringe is not something we like to see when we visit the doctor. McLean bravely likens injecting insulin to brushing her teeth. She is bold to make such a claim, because if I were brushing my teeth in front of you, you wouldn't think twice. If, however, I pulled out a syringe and injected myself, you might wonder what was going on. What I am trying to point out here is that often how others see a person with diabetes can stigmatize the condition further.

On November 4, 1992 the *Langley Times* ran a front-page feature article on type 1 diabetes. The photo showed a little girl injecting insulin into her arm, leaning with her arm against a windowpane to make a mound of skin—a realistic photo of a child with diabetes who was treating her condition. Some time after the article ran, the paper printed a letter to the editor which spoke volumes as to just how misguided and misinformed people are in relation to diabetes. A woman wrote to say how upset she was about the front-page photo of the little girl using a needle. She was concerned that children may "find used needles in the bushes and use them."

I have never read of any reported circumstance of children finding needles in suburban bushes and using them. That's much more of a concern in the inner city, where heroin addicts litter the street with syringes and leave them in elementary school playgrounds.

Despite the misinformation in the original article (which I'll touch on later), the picture spoke many more words. Indeed, the photo hopefully promoted healthy discussion about the reality of diabetes in a little girl's life. To censor it would be completely counterproductive.

Strangely, there is a mythic association in the public's mind between needles and drug addicts. So where should one take an insulin shot without provoking a disturbance?

Though I hate the addict association, it may be useful to illustrate that the person with diabetes may start to think like a junkie—looking for a place to shoot up around meal times and plagued by social stigma. With my experiences of having to give a syringe full of insulin at least twice daily, I have discovered, remarkably, that it does not really matter where you are. Privacy is nice, but not necessary. It is better to give it in a crowded restaurant than not to give it at all, right?

This puts the person with diabetes in a rather awkward situation. I find people are too absorbed in their own affairs to really care that a person right beside them is injecting a substance into themselves. There are those with diabetes who choose to hide their condition from the world—sometimes as a justified survival mechanism—and others who choose not to hide it at all.

Don't feel responsible for other people's reactions. They probably don't understand what it's all about. Why feel ashamed? Early on I did feel anxiety that I had to perform this activity in public, but now I'm quite good at it. I can draw insulin from two bottles and be finished in a matter of seconds, and if people ask questions, let them. Speak to them about it. It takes a lot of energy and courage, but awareness fares better than ignorance.

Driving Me Crazy

Diabetes and driving raises a host of controversial issues. The most common worry is the possibility of a low blood sugar reaction (hypoglycemia) while driving.

On the fateful day of June 18, 1996, I received a driver's medical exam, which said I had to have a "routine" physical for a "known medical disability."

Now that was news to me—the idea that I should take time off work to go to a doctor's office for an unnecessary physical when I was perfectly healthy.

I wrote a letter to the then B.C. Minister of Transportation and Highways, Lois Boone. The letter, dated June 23, 1996, raised three points. First, that the medical exam was a waste of my time and money. Second, that diabetes had never affected my driving skills, and third, that the Motor Vehicle Branch was discriminating against healthy people that happened to have a chronic illness such as diabetes. I asked to have the medical exam waived, considering the nature of my condition.

On September 16, 1996 I received a letter from C.J. Morris, who was the Superintendent of Motor Vehicles, saying my immediate action was necessary, so I immediately wrote another letter along the same theme as the Lois Boone letter.

While I did not receive a response to the C.J. Morris letter, I did receive a response on December 2, 1996 from Vicki Farrally, who was the Assistant Deputy Minister. After apologizing for the lengthy delay, she quoted the statutes of the Motor Vehicle Act. What disturbed me was the assumption of diabetes as a "risk that may endanger the driver or anyone else." According to Ms. Farrally, the Motor Vehicle Branch had the "statutory responsibility to determine the fitness and ability of an individual to safely operate a vehicle." This standard of fitness is assessed through the British Columbia Medical Association. Not surprisingly, Ms. Farrally wrote that my "continued fitness to drive must be evaluated through periodic medical reports completed by (my) physician."

With this excuse, the case seemed closed.

Unfortunately, the letter did not address the fact that many people with diabetes are perfectly healthy and are in no way unfit to drive. In fact, there are people who are driving at this very moment who are definitely unfit to drive and are not asked to complete a physical. This is the challenge of confronting entrenched government bureaucracies and hypocrites.

As I did not receive a response to C.J. Morris' letter and had since lost the medical examination because of the delay, I did not have a medical exam. I wasn't too concerned because I was riding my bike to and from work every day, so did not require a license to operate a motor vehicle.

That was, of course, until September 30, 1998. Reacting with the characteristic speed of government (two years), a mean-spirited letter revoking my license ended up in my mailbox. Without any warning and without any further letters, the government decided to act and force me to have my medical exam or damn the world. They decided that I must have some sort of reason for delaying the exam so long, so Mark Medgyesi, Superintendent of Motor Vehicles, decided to pull my license because I had not had a physical.

Weighing my options with the threat of imprisonment and

fines if I drove without a license, I phoned and I heard the broken record again, in case I forgot that to the Motor Vehicle Branch I had a "known medical disability" and needed to have a medical exam even though I was completely healthy. In fact, they added, they can force someone to have an exam at any time if they think that person can't drive because of his or her medical condition.

I took time off work, thereby losing pay. I paid $40 to the doctor for a physical I didn't need, only to have the doctor write "Well controlled diabetes HbA1c 0.068 Jan./98. Rare hypo-glycemia—not severe—no impairment of consciousness."

At least I was supporting the medical system.

It then got me to wondering just how many of these unnec-essary exams were being demanded, compared to actual acci-dents caused by those with diabetes. It also got me to thinking what a defensive driver I am and that there are many people without diabetes on the road driving that should not be.

I submitted a comment regarding this discrimination via the Premier's Youth Office because I was not satisfied with the answers I'd received. On December 30, 1998, I received another bureaucratic response, which was the most eloquently written, from Lisa Howie, Director of Driver Fitness. Hers was a much more detailed response, saying that a follow-up medical exam was required one year after diagnosis and every five years there-after. Diabetes is a "progressive" condition. I had never thought of it that way before:

> As our records do not contain any medical information regarding the severity, progression, treatment or effects of your medical condition, diabetes mellitus, it is neces-sary that you submit a completed medical report. As each individual is affected by diabetes differently and diabetes is a progressive condition, this medical information will provide the assurance that you have remained medically fit to operate a motor vehicle safely.

The Driver's Medical Examination requirement is enabled

under the authority of section 29 of the Motor Vehicle Act, which she quoted in her letter:

> The superintendent may require a person to whom a driver's license has been issued to attend at a time and place for one or both of the following purposes:
>   (a) To submit to one or more of the following tests, to be conducted by the Insurance Corporation of British Columbia: a knowledge test; a road test; a road signs and signals test;
>   (b) To be otherwise examined as to the person's fitness and ability to drive and operate motor vehicles of the category for which he or she is licensed. [18]

That letter was supposed to shut me up. I had a disability that might impair my driving ability. I would be judged on an individual basis, along with all others with diabetes. That's a lot of unnecessary medicals. That's a lot of money.

As I said before, despite the Motor Vehicle Act, there are people who are driving on the road who do not have diabetes and should not be driving. Perhaps policing sitting ducks, such as those who have admitted truthfully to the Motor Vehicle Branch that they have diabetes, is easier than actually policing the actions that kill people, such as drinking and driving, road rage and speeding?

It's almost enough to make you want to conceal the fact that you even have the condition in the first place, so as not to be treated differently. But for me, it was too late for that, and I don't recommend lying to governement offices. But I know people with diabetes who haven't volunteered the information because of things just like this.

I don't have much faith in government processes. Government, in effect, discriminates against a minority of the population with diabetes who are no more prone to dangerous driver fitness than the next person. (I didn't know there was a director of driver fitness. Do they make people get out of their cars at stoplights and do a few jumping jacks?)

I believe people with diabetes should take responsibility for their actions the same as anyone else. If someone is drunk, drives and causes an accident, they should have their license revoked. If someone is having a low blood sugar, drives and causes an accident, they should have their license revoked. Though I suppose if the Motor Vehicle Branch could, they would issue physicals to all those who drink alcohol, just to make sure they're no danger to themselves or other drivers. How much taxpayer money is wasted on such campaigns? Having a serious insulin reaction while driving is a danger. But realistically speaking, if I am having a reaction, I will not drive. Just as if I have taken some cold medication that makes me drowsy, I will not operate heavy machinery.

Choosing not to drive at all is a realistic choice for some. When I worked downtown in Vancouver, I rode my bicycle both ways—it was refreshing not having to pay for car insurance and gasoline. Not having a driver's license doesn't matter if you ride a bike. Riding a bike, you develop a greater appreciation for the dangers of motorized vehicles, and the psychotic driving methods of many people who don't have to take medical exams every few years to see if they're fit to narrowly miss hitting cyclists and pedestrians.

Flying With Diabetes

Eileen Bahlsen was the first person in the world with type 1 diabetes to be licensed to fly an aircraft solo. That's solo—without any safety pilot. Before April 1992, anyone who wanted a pilot's license had to obtain a medical certificate, which was not granted to people with type 1 diabetes.

On June 10, 1991, Eileen was told she was "medically unfit to hold any form of flight-crew license." On November 4, she launched a Federal Court case against this blanket restriction, claiming that it violated her rights under section 15 of the Canadian Charter of Rights and Freedoms. Eileen realized that she was not being considered on an individual basis and that if she were, she'd be seen as fit to hold the license. Justice

Frederick Gibson agreed. On June 30, 1995, the federal court judge declared the regulation was against the Canadian Charter of Rights and Freedoms, and therefore was of no force or effect.

The American Diabetes Association became embroiled in a similar struggle for pilot Daryl Williams. The Federal Aviation Administration (FAA) denied anyone with insulin-treated diabetes a certificate that would allow a person to pilot a plane. Daryl Williams had qualified for a commercial as well as a private pilot's license, until he developed diabetes.

The FAA's blanket ban denied a medical certificate to those who required insulin injections. The ban did not stop Daryl from piloting a plane with another pilot on board.

In 1991, the American Diabetes Association filed a petition with the FAA that asked them to drop its blanket restriction. It also asked that each pilot be considered as an individual. Through letter-writing campaigns, a protocol written by endocrinologists and many organizations including the Juvenile Diabetes Research Foundation, The Aircraft Owners and Pilots Association, and the American Association of Diabetes Educators, history was in the making.

It took medical professionals to join in the struggle before the petition was considered seriously. In December 1996, after a full five years of convincing, the FAA dropped its policy, taking the protocol seriously. Those with type 1 diabetes could be evaluated on an individual basis at last.

People with diabetes have the ability to oppose unjust blanket restrictions and blatant discrimination. Eileen Bahlsen and Daryl Williams did it and so can you. It just takes a lot of time, perseverance and money for lawyers.

Chapter 7
Travelling With Diabetes

Before the Trip

Before you take that trip down to Mexico, there are a few things that will make the travelling experience run smoothly. Scheduling a visit with the doctor before the trip is crucial—besides getting a check up and possible vaccines if you're travelling to risk areas, make sure you discuss changing time zones and the changes in insulin times and meal planning. Be sure to work out a schedule with your doctor when determining dosages for the flight.

Be sure also to get a letter that says you require insulin, syringes and other supplies to treat diabetes. This will help if a customs officer finds your syringes and suspects the worst—something, I might add, that has not happened to me despite all the borders I've crossed. It can't hurt, though.

There was a customs officer in Heathrow (the main airport in London) who asked me about my syringes. The conversation that followed was not intended to put me on the defensive—the officer had seen those with diabetes pass through customs before—but was a subtle way to verify the presence of these items. He asked me how long I'd had diabetes, whether I took insulin and if the machine they'd seen in the X-ray was a blood-testing meter. (He mentioned later that diabetes was in his family too, which made me think that diabetes has touched many different people around the world.)

Health insurance is also a worthwhile investment for the time you'll be travelling. Make sure it covers people with diabetes. Some still don't.

Travel Survival Checklist

Here is a checklist of useful things to take related to diabetes:

- Double the amount of diabetes supplies that you'll need for the trip
- Extra snacks in case of delayed meals
- Extra sugar sources for low blood sugar including juice tetra packs, dried fruit, candy, et cetera
- Glucagon kit and ketone strips
- First aid kit
- Extra battery for blood glucose meter
- Medic Alert ID saying you have diabetes
- Comfortable shoes

If I had not brought an extra supply of insulin when I travelled to Mazatlan, Mexico, I would have had to come back to Canada and cut my trip short. Why? I dropped an insulin bottle on the tiled floor of the hotel and it smashed into a million pieces. Always bring an extra bottle or two, or you may find yourself seriously stuck.

Snacks and sugar sources are common sense—it's not fun getting low because an airline promised dinner and all you got was a stale package of pretzels. Be sure not to depend on airlines and hotels to supply food if you need it.

In my travels I've never taken a glucagon kit and ketone strips, even though I've put them on the checklist. This comes down to choices. I don't regret the decision because I've never needed either of them, though they could come in handy in an unfortunate emergency, such as if you're travelling to an area where there is no doctor for miles around.

Why not pop those sandals off and go running in the surf on

the beach in Mazatlan? Choices again. Oh, I have diabetes and must protect my feet, you say? Little cuts might lead to infections, particularly if you don't feel the little cuts or ignore them. Foot infections are the leading cause of amputations today for those with diabetes.

True, protecting your feet is important, but I find it hard to wear shoes on a beach. Mine stay off, and I tend to enjoy swimming better without them. In hindsight, however, maybe I could have taken more precautions to protect my feet in Mexico. If I cut my foot somehow, there would not have been adequate medical treatment there.

Just be careful. That's all anybody can ask. That's why I added a first aid kit to my list.

Another useful thing to have when travelling is a Medic Alert bracelet. If an emergency happens, the medics will see the bracelet and realize that you have diabetes. I struggled with this, because it does label you as having a medical condition, and people inevitably ask questions about it. But especially when travelling, it's crucial, because you're somewhere that might be unfamiliar. If you suffer a low blood sugar, for instance, no one will know what to do unless you tell them.

Always bring extra food. The times I arrived at my destination with no stores around open late at night would have been worse if I had no food packed. I try to plan as if I won't receive any food whatsoever, so I'll always have some sort of supply. Never assume that you'll be served that in-flight dinner or that the hotel restaurant will be open. Things get delayed. Your baggage may end up in Timbuktu. There might be an outbreak of salmonella poisoning and everything might be closed. In some places, food is really hard to come by if you're arriving late at night and everything's closed.

Transporting Insulin

Keep insulin and all diabetes supplies on you at all times in your carry-on luggage, to make sure they don't disappear or end up in Madrid when you're in London. This is another reason you have the letter written by the doctor, in case you have to visit the pharmacy to obtain some emergency supplies.

Insulin does not need to be kept cold; it is actually stable at body temperature. So why do pharmacies refrigerate insulin? As a precaution, presumably, because it's supposed to make it last longer. (Of course, this doesn't help much if the temperature where you're going gets super hot.) Refrigerated, insulin will last until the printed expiry date on the box. At room temperature, it lasts several months, and at body temperature, it lasts a few weeks. Freezing and temperatures that are higher than body temperature destroy insulin. One of the best ways to cook a bottle of insulin, and thus render it unusable, is to leave it in a closed car when the sun is out. I'm speaking from experience here.

If you're visiting a tropical destination or are concerned about a possible lack of refrigeration, try to keep insulin cold by any means possible. I bought a portable lunch box cooler that kept things cool with a frozen gel pack in it. Some other ways to keep it cold include: ice, a cool wet cloth, or frozen food (sealed) to use as cold pack.

Be sure to keep an eye on your insulin supply. If anything looks strange—for example, if clumps appear, if what was once clear becomes cloudy or if the bottle gets broken—dispose of it. By tracking blood sugar, you are more likely to notice that something's not right, because an unexplained gradual increase in blood sugars could be a sign that insulin has gone bad.

In Mexico I would descend the adobe steps to the beach-side bar to fill up a pitcher of ice. I used the Spanish word for ice (*hielo*) every morning in my Anglicized Spanish. I then left the insulin in a bag in the pitcher. On returning after one fine day in the Mazatlan sun, I was horrified to see the pitcher missing.

I asked my wife if she'd seen it. She replied no. We searched the whole hotel room for it, but the pitcher was gone. This could very well have cut the trip short. Then I saw a maid with a cart changing some towels. I asked her about it and she said she'd thrown it out. I said that it contained some important medicine for me and she actually found it—I don't know where it had been. After washing it off (it had still been in the sealed bag), it was all right, luckily.

When I was in Spain—Barcelona specifically—there was no refrigeration at the campsite we were staying at. Being resourceful, I went to the camp grocery store and found a wide assortment of Spanish frozen foods. Of all the frozen foods I tried (peas, corn, crab, among others), corn worked the best, only because it was packaged in small bags that were sealed. It doesn't work very well if it's an open bag that leaks when thawing, making the insulin bottles all slimy.

I was quite lucky through most of the seven months of European travel because I brought two frozen gel packs; when one had thawed, I'd usually be able to find a freezer somewhere. In Toledo, for instance, I asked if I could use the freezer at a campsite market. The answer was no, because they couldn't exactly keep track of everyone's food. I said it was so I could keep my medicine cold and they changed their mind. Each morning, I'd switch the frozen gel packs, keeping the insulin cool in the stifling heat. Sometimes people are more congenial when it's framed as a life-and-death issue—as it should be.

Syringe and Lancet Disposal

Even though disposable syringes say "use once and destroy," they can be reused, as can lancets. Be sure to take precautions, however, such as recapping both ends and discarding if it's been dropped, looks dirty or is damaged (if the needle is bent, for example). If it's uncomfortable to inject, dispose of the syringe too, because its protective silicon coating has possibly worn off. Be sure not to wipe the needle with alcohol, as this will remove the silicon coating.

Most of the same goes for lancets. In my experience, I reused syringes because I found it a waste to dispose of them when they could be reused again. I did, however, take double the amount I needed along on the seven-month trip to Europe, which meant fourteen months of syringes, lancets and blood sugar test strips.

For syringe and lancet disposal, the best way is to clip the needles off so that they don't poke anybody while in the garbage. I used my Swiss army knife to cut the needles off. Be sure not to prick yourself. You can buy a device for to collect the cut s, but I used a vitamin pill container or a medicine container. These can be taken to a medical waste facility.

In Case of Emergency

If you're facing an emergency, be sure to seek medical treatment immediately. Make sure you contact your medical insurance company as soon as possible to confirm treatment; sometimes they require you fly back to the country of origin if that's possible.

The Canadian or American consulates can help when abroad. As for treatment, university hospitals are more likely to have a diabetes specialist on staff. If you can't find a doctor, the International Association for Medical Assistance (phone 716-754-4883) can refer you to a doctor abroad.

Chapter 8
More From the Front Line

No Day Off

Diabetes is exhausting, and exhaustion, intensified through day after day of blood tests, insulin injections, dietary considerations and exercise, can lead to burnout.

A vacation would be great; or maybe just a day off. There is no day off with diabetes, but imagine the pressure that would be relieved to be able to forget about diabetes, even for just one day. Sleep in without a worry, wake up and eat a hearty breakfast—any food you'd like, of course—go to the beach, jump into the water, and swim through the lapping waves with not a care in the world. Insulin? What's that? Eat food? Only when I feel hungry. Schedule? Who needs it? Cut my foot on the coral reef? I just need a plastic bandage—it's no big deal.

Doing whatever you like to do best without a setback, no limits—flying a plane through clear blue sky, perhaps, or boating around on the ocean.

Spending time with people, maybe having a party, playing some volleyball in the sand and inviting everybody over for dinner, because you could forget about lunch—you aren't hungry—only to have dinner later in the night on the beach to the sound of deep rhythms of music. Of course, by this time you're hungry and eat anything you'd like at the buffet on the beach, perhaps having a few drinks without a care and laughing.

Going to bed late, in the wee hours of the morning, after

dancing to your favourite music under the stars and seeing the constellations move across the sky, feeling at one with the universe, knowing that life is fine and nothing's wrong and nothing is there to spoil it.

Sure, it's a fantasy. But you can always dream.

I'm not so sure that the idyllic bubble wouldn't burst anyway. Maybe there'd be salmonella poisoning because the food wasn't cooked properly. Maybe it would rain on the beach, forcing everyone to huddle in leaky condos. Perhaps people would start singing really awful karaoke songs.

Sometimes we think that a day off from life would be helpful, but no matter what problems assail us, our lives are still our lives and we can't hide from them. It takes courage to become who you really are and not develop wild neuroses. There's no day off from diabetes, so learn to laugh at it, right in the face.

Morality Play

The public perception of diabetes is influenced by our personal testimonies. We have portrayed a disease that is no more than a minor inconvenience. It is little wonder that when things go wrong we are accused of noncompliance, mismanagement, and "cheating" on diets... By showing the world only the happy face, and not the tragic disease beneath, we are endorsing the prevailing philosophy of tolerating, rather than curing, diabetes. [19]

As Deb Butterfield suggests, diabetes magazines that show healthy people managing their condition with the strength and vigor of a hard-core athlete send a mixed message. It's not only the nonprofits who illustrate that actual people (and often superhuman people) have diabetes, but also pharmaceutical companies who show shiny happy people with the latest blood glucose meter or syringe. Although it is not crippling, diabetes is more than a minor inconvenience.

Often, if complications develop, the person with diabetes is blamed for his or her behaviour. Sometimes he or she is even blamed for developing the condition in the first place. Because, according to Kristine Alster:

> Health is held among the highest of values and is believed to be a state achievable by right acts and sufficient will, illness ceases to be a misfortune and is taken as evidence of moral failing. [20]

Blame only serves to neglect the reality of the complexities of managing the condition, involving routine, diet and insulin, and other fears of social isolation, disability and death. Diabetes is unsettling because it "...calls into question plans, expectations, habits, goals, one's image of one's life, and even life itself." [21]

However irrational the blame, even physicians descend into the moralistic language of the "good" versus "bad" diabetic; for example, by accusing a patient of "cheating." Guilt is an extremely damaging way to make a patient compliant, and casting blame does not help to turn people to the good side. People with diabetes become stigmatized when behaviour is judged in a moralistic way; for instance, by doctors who attach an almost mythical significance to a particular Hemoglobin A1c result. The test itself is seen as "good" or "bad," and these judgments are then cast on the patient.

The Hemoglobin A1c (HbA1c) is a test that measures overall blood glucose control over a number of months. Too often, however, this "measure of health status is used as a substitute measure of behaviour." [22] Ludicrously, a doctor will assume that a patient hasn't complied with his or her prescription. If the HbA1c is high, the assumption is that the patient has failed in some miserable way to do something within his or her control. If the HbA1c is in the "normal" range, all is well. This measurement is sadly inadequate as it reduces the complexity of the whole individual to one test.

It follows that if blood sugars are labelled "good" or "bad," then the person himself is labeled a "good" or "bad" person with diabetes, in what is an extremely damaging morality play. In fact, it's not a moralistic thing. Blood sugars are not good or bad, and if you would like to apply such labels, it's "good" that you're testing in the first place to see what your blood sugar is. There are people who have impeccable blood sugar control and are shocked when they develop the complications of diabetes. They should not be blamed for the unpredictable consequences of their condition.

Much of life is about challenging our bodily boundaries. Living with diabetes challenges a boundary. This is heroic.

Complications of the Diabetes Control and Complications Trial (DCCT)

The Diabetes Control and Complications Trial (DCCT) was a much-lauded study conducted from 1983 to 1993 to determine the effects of "intensive" versus "conventional" insulin therapy. Intensive therapy consisted of more than three injections of insulin a day or insulin pump therapy; four or more blood tests a day; dietary instruction; and monthly visits to medical professionals. Conventional therapy, however, consisted of one or two injections a day; visits with medical professionals every three months; and daily urine or blood testing. The National Institutes of Health (NIH) in the United States spent some $280 million [23] on this study, which proved conclusively that those with diabetes should test blood sugar and attempt to maintain a normal blood sugar.

In the intensive group, low blood sugar occurred three times as much as in the conventional group. They also gained more weight (presumably from the extra food to treat the more frequent low blood sugars) than the conventional group. While the study did focus on diabetes management, it did not prove conclusively that complications wouldn't develop even if blood sugars were controlled. It did, however, say that the chances were better if you managed the daily challenge of insulin, diet and blood tests.

Unfortunately, the DCCT also shifted the focus of blame. Those with diabetes were blamed for developing complications, despite the fact that insulin therapy, however religiously followed, does not guarantee a life free of complications. [24] Diabetes is the problem, not the people who have it.

Deb Butterfield, in her book *Showdown With Diabetes*, puts it this way:

> People who live with insulin-dependent diabetes know that good blood-sugar control is better than poor blood-sugar control, but although insulin, glucose tests, diets, and exercise are *necessary* to manage diabetes, they are by no means *sufficient*. Some people need only moderately good blood-sugar control to prevent complications; others need perfect control, but as the DCCT showed, perfect control is rarely achieved—even with intensive insulin therapy. [25]

What Butterfield means is that control is important, but lifestyle changes and diabetes management skills are not necessarily sufficient to control blood sugar levels. Other factors besides food, insulin and exercise must be taken into consideration. These include, "...stress, excitement, delayed meals, meals in restaurants, travel, infections, colds, unscheduled activities, and of course, adolescence," [26] not to mention menstrual cycles, and other factors that are often unidentifiable and unexplainable. The likelihood of complications is also a question of genetic susceptibility.

While it seems like the DCCT is the be-all and end-all of research in the diabetes area, it is worth noting that intensive blood glucose control is not without its disadvantages. Intensive treatment patients gained an average of ten pounds more weight and experienced more frequent severe hypoglycemic reactions. On the other hand, the results found complications were reduced considerably with intensive therapy over standard therapy.

The DCCT cost millions of dollars and was the largest study in diabetes history, but one could argue that it did not directly help people with diabetes. Many who had diabetes couldn't understand the priorities of investing in a study that was not focused on finding a cure for diabetes. Those with diabetes had already been testing their blood sugars, and with the DCCT, nothing changed what was already known.

Those with consistently "normal" blood sugar levels are unlikely to have complications at all. This is because they don't have diabetes. Having high and low blood sugar levels is the definition of diabetes; this brings the whole point of the DCCT into question.

One might also question the involvement of the 43 pharmaceutical companies who provided diabetes supplies in "generous support" of the DCCT, suggesting the high interest of these companies in diabetes management research funded by U.S. federal medical research funds. It's also interesting to note that:

• No minority groups were represented in the DCCT, though many groups suffer a higher incidence of diabetes than do caucasians.
• There were few teens involved, even though diabetes is often diagnosed in adolescence.
• The intensive therapy group had a level of care that would be extremely difficult if not impossible to maintain in day-to-day life (i.e., they had their own team adjusting multiple doses of insulin, they tested their blood sugar frequently, they ate a restricted diet at proper times and followed an exercise regimen). [27]

There is no guarantee that complications will not develop, even with intensive insulin therapy and blood sugar monitoring. It is, however, less likely that they will, which is sufficient reason to keep tabs on diabetes. Still, there is a genetic factor that is often overlooked in the equation—the possibility of developing complications is bound up in a genetic predisposition. This explains why some people live long lives with diabetes without complications, while others experience complications more frequently.

Although I haven't talked much about the complications of

diabetes, there is really only one "serious" complication to any medical condition: death. No matter how much plastic surgery you have or how many doctors are trying to keep you alive, everybody will die eventually. Death is a part of life that Western medicine seems bent on destroying at any cost, even if it sometimes means sacrificing quality of life.

I know people with diabetes who are immaculately healthy, and I also know people with diabetes who have severe complications. Both agree that complications are not necessarily in the control of the person with diabetes. If complications are going to develop, it's part of the process, just as death is a natural part of life.

What we can be optimistic about are the advances in diabetes management. We can test blood sugars more accurately; inject insulin, such as lispro insulin, that is even more like the normal functioning of the pancreas; and we can use an insulin pump that is only as big as a credit card.

Unfortunately, the morality play continues. Consider the following questions posed by Jerry Edelwich and Archie Brodsky in their book *Diabetes: Caring for Your Emotions as well as Your Health*:

> Does going a certain number of years without complications (mean) good conduct or a good constitution? Should a person who does not have diabetes be rewarded for having a pancreas that secretes insulin? [28]

Of course not—the idea is ludicrous. The issue is complex, but the DCCT in 1993 suggested that tighter control meant less of a chance of complications later in life. The choices that need to be made are often lifestyle choices, such as what a person eats at what times.

Unfortunately, the benefits of intensive therapy do not rule out the possibility of future complications, and low blood sugars and weight gain are unappealing side effects. A happy medium between conventional and intensive therapy is all that can be expected.

Suicide

Ernest Hemingway had diabetes. He also committed suicide. I don't consider him to be a very good role model in that regard.

A friend of mine committed suicide a while back. He was the president of the Canadian Diabetes Association youth group, and a role model for me. We had a similar sense of humour, enjoying Monty Python movies and just hanging out. He needed the group more than anyone else. We looked to him for leadership, but all along it was really him who needed support. It has been said that people who are the most outgoing and successful are sometimes the most insecure inside. They don't allow their true feelings to surface because they are too afraid of getting hurt. My friend and I lost touch over the years, and I don't know what happened or why he did it. It's probably a question that can never be answered.

I still think about him a lot. It's been years since it happened, but he'll always be with me. He was a part of my life and had touched many others through his volunteer work. He was a person with diabetes.

Obviously, it's not only diabetes that can trigger suicidal impulses. Parental problems, relationship fights and peer pressure sometimes make one feel like it's all not worth it, but a chronic disease doesn't make things seem any brighter. Surviving with diabetes takes a lot of courage, and anyone should be proud of doing it—it's certainly not easy. Diabetes may add another dimension to someone's personal struggles, because it may seem like there is no way out. The threat of suicide needs to be taken seriously.

Part of the problem may be that people with diabetes often feel isolated by their condition. I thought I was alone with diabetes when I was first diagnosed. I wish I knew then what I know now. It's a humbling experience, and a challenge physically and emotionally.

A woman with diabetes I once knew decided that, somehow, she had been selected to die by nature and was now living on borrowed time. If she lived in the wilderness, she argued, she would die, without a doubt. But so would most people if they were uprooted from a life in the city to fend for themselves in a wilderness environment. She tried to rationalize her suicidal wishes, suggesting that she was supposed to die and that surviving wasn't natural.

I sometimes feel as if I, too, am living on borrowed time, but I disagreed with her. Humankind has a natural instinct for self-preservation. Surviving with diabetes is entirely natural. It is natural to inject insulin and to survive. It is natural for a human being to want to stay alive and live life to the fullest.

Here is a poem, the original version of which I wrote on March 9, 1992. At this time I was very angry about diabetes and was trying to figure out what I was going to do with my life. I had broken up with my girlfriend at the time and was exploring the depths of depression. The feelings I had around diabetes were brought up in full force, and I had time to reflect on how diabetes was affecting my life.

Bloodlet
I as "diabetic": person as disorder
in a pancreatic prison.

Plastic syringes,
pincushion fingers,
applying pressure to obtain beads of sweet blood.
Testing blood glucose, counting days,
obsessively recording doctored results.

No crimson fluid appears today,
though I am sure blood percolates through my veins
seen every day through capillary fingers,
tough skinned
calloused layers resist entry.

Complicated, comatose,
crippled by capillaries,
bleeding blood vessel eyes,
like King Lear.

Normal people productive, predictable,
choking on clocked hours,
like dark nightmares without faces,
abnormal pages of fashion magazines,
post-modern plastic Barbie exhibitionist
individualistic,
in solitary confinement.

A ritualistic normal life of blood tests,
insulin injections,
exercise and diet,
textbooks of doctors and dietitians,
lab technicians and ophthalmologists.

Stabbing still reveals no blood,
blunt lancet finding frozen fingers.

Sometimes ink fails to flow freely
like blood,
mouths are taped shut
in solitary desperation,
bound and gagged by clocks,
syringes, and blood.

I have been angry for many years about diabetes. I have never accepted diabetes, but I live with it. I still have angry moments, but had to learn how to channel the anger in more productive ways. Like writing this book.

Diabetes is a do-or-die situation, and I think people forget that when they see people with diabetes who look healthy and in top form. Sure, we don't want to dwell on feeling sorry for ourselves, but it's a stage that we must overcome to become fully human and be able to live with diabetes, even if we cannot accept it.

Part Three
INSTITUTIONAL DIABETES

Chapter 9
The Nonprofit Organization Experience

Canadian Diabetes Association (CDA): My Experience

We spend hundreds of millions of dollars each year on diabetes nonprofit organizations. Much of this is used for diabetes research, but I often find myself asking the question, Where does the rest of this money go?

Insulin might be considered one of the most lifesaving discoveries of the twentieth century, but it's interesting to note that the discovery was made on a hunch by the Canadian Fred Banting, who was by no means an expert scientist in his field, or funded by nonprofit organizations or pharmaceutical companies. The discovery of insulin is shrouded in mystery and intrigue, but they just got really lucky, borrowing a University of Toronto lab and testing on many dogs that died in the process. Banting teamed up with Charles Best, who went on to found the Canadian Diabetes Association (CDA).

I first encountered the CDA in 1989, just after my diagnosis-day ordeal in the hospital. At the time I was looking to meet others who were living with diabetes.

Educational pamphlets, which were rather outdated and missed the mark entirely with regards to my age group, sketched my first picture of the CDA as an organization that was supposed to be there for those with diabetes. I found out about a youth group that met at the CDA office, where other peers with type 1 diabetes met.

I never would have gone, but a man named Don Black convinced me to give it a shot. He was the president of the CDA youth group at the time, and he wanted me to come to the meeting to check it out. He smoked, had a cool car and tended to drive faster than he should have, but I didn't mind one bit. He was someone I looked up to.

That fateful night I decided to go to the meeting, just to check out what they were all about. I didn't expect too much, so I wouldn't be disappointed if it was a disaster. It took a lot of courage, first of all to admit to strangers that I had diabetes—considering I was fresh out of the hospital—and second, to take such a long trip from Langley into Vancouver to meet at the CDA office.

The group was intended for youth who had diabetes but was open to whomever else wanted to show up. I met people my age who had been through a lot of what I was experiencing and who seemed normal and alive. The youth group did foster a sense of belonging, each of us knowing exactly why we were there and sharing tips. They were warm meetings in a cold environment, an artificial office space that did not lend itself to informal meetings. There were some shared stories of difficult ordeals with diabetes, unofficial tips on diabetes management, and a sense of understanding of what each of us was going through. We were a group of people meeting around a common issue and with a common goal.

The youth group was involved in a fundraiser for the CDA

"Support" Group Stigma

Some people have problems with the concept of "support" groups, perhaps because the demand to be individually healthy impairs our ability to remain compassionate to others. In fact, I doubt anyone can do it alone. Believe me, I've tried.

Support groups aren't only a sounding board for people who complain about all their ailments and the depressing aspects of diabetes. They are there to help people deal with change and get on and I ended up volunteering to put up posters. At the same time, I was living in Langley and was still attending high school, so the commute to the CDA office in Vancouver was long and tedious.

Through my brief experience with the youth group, I learned a lot about people, especially that others beside myself could cope with a chronic condition. Diabetes was an awful point of similarity between immensely different people. We had parties, watched movies, ate pizza and hung out, but it started to dwindle, and when the president stepped down, it completely unravelled. Don was the glue holding the group together.

In 1991, while the group was still operating, I had the fortunate opportunity to be vice president of the group. We had the addresses and phone numbers of 500 people in the Lower Mainland who were registered youth members of the CDA. A handful of dedicated members still attended regular meetings and were active in the events that we planned.

We submitted a budget to the CDA, with the hopes of resuscitating the already dwindling group. The CDA came through with some money, but despite having a budget, nothing seemed enough to convince people with diabetes to attend the meetings. Indeed, many people with diabetes, including myself, have a bad taste in their mouth left by the CDA, for reasons I will discuss later in this chapter.

After Don's departure, we tried to keep the group going. It still baffles me why the youth group fell apart. It was something I wanted to exist. It was something that people did need, despite

---

with their lives. It's also a way to see how others deal with diabetes.

There are many groups that don't necessarily call themselves "support" groups but fulfill that role in people's lives in much the same way. Playing softball every week during the summer, volunteering for Meals on Wheels or working in an animal shelter are just some examples of ways people can get involved with their community and forget about their troubles for a moment, even if it isn't directly related to diabetes.

the lack of attendance. Was it a case of collective denial? Perhaps it was the nature of diabetes: Who would want to admit in their teens that they had a chronic condition and participate in events that might set them apart from the norm?

We phoned those 500 youth members of the CDA, campaigned, set up fundraisers, and had trips and activities ready to go. Our telemarketing campaign assault on the CDA list brought many promises to come out to the meetings, but in the end we had too many empty chairs, which was discouraging. Other ideas were put forward; we even created and published a youth group newsletter called *The Funky Chicken* to stir up interest, but to no avail. There were only a handful of responses.

Soon after, the group dissolved. I have no knowledge of any successful CDA youth group. This is very unfortunate as it means there is little in the way of support for teenagers with diabetes who may be feeling alone at a vitally important time in their lives. Starting one takes time, energy and a very good sense of humour, though it can be done.

As a result of my youth group experience, I came to face the fact that the CDA is ill-equipped to reach those with type 1 diabetes. It focuses almost solely on type 2 diabetes (90 percent of the diabetes population), because the CDA must meet the demands of their membership. Those with type 1 diabetes are, ironically, marginalized by the very organization that is supposed to offer them support and solace. It is also strongly focused on Ontario. The CDA's Eastern Canadian bias is a reality that is reflected in the structure of many nonprofit organizations in Canada.

Another unfortunate reality is the frequency of turnover that exists at the CDA. All the people I knew years ago have moved on, and many people use the CDA as a stepping stone to bigger, better jobs. Hey, that's fine for some, but for an organization that deals with people who have a chronic condition, it would be better if there were more of an ongoing connection to the people it's supposed to serve.

The CDA's mission is to "promote the health of Canadians through diabetes research, education, services and advocacy."

According to their fact sheet, the CDA spends 32 percent of its funding on research, 30 percent on services, 16 percent on education and 5 percent on advocacy. After my initial experience with outdated and irrelevant CDA pamphlets that were given to me at the hospital, I don't believe education is the CDA's strong suit. While it's clear that the general public needs to be educated about diabetes, people with diabetes need an organization that will serve as a support system for their whole lives and will fight on behalf of their rights. People who are involved with CDA need to believe in its values and advocate for people with diabetes.

Disease of the Month Club

November is Diabetes Month. In fact, each month has its associate disease—you could go a full year focusing on each ailment known to humanity. I find it odd that nonprofits would promote this concept, each year gearing up for a big publicity run during the month. For me, diabetes is year round.

When the article in the *Langley Times* with the photo of the girl injecting herself during Diabetes Month in 1992, I nearly wept with joy, as everyone who saw the paper had to confront an intimate moment in this girl's life. I read the article avidly, delighted that the plight was publicized to this extent, illustrating the ongoing struggle with diabetes from the front page on.

At the time, I had never really questioned media. The TV, radio and newspaper were, to me, mere recorders of historical fact. They were the purveyors of objectivity and unbiased news reporting and investigative journalism, right? Not exactly.

My first real experience with the misinformation promoted through mass media laid the foundation for my future studies at university in communications, dissecting inner workings of media ownership, content and form.

The *Times* article contained gross errors regarding diabetes management. I was appalled at the inaccuracies and enraged, reading the sloppily written article over and over again, disbelieving what I read. I wrote a letter to the editor of the *Langley Times*, which appeared on November 14, 1992, under the headline "Diabetes Turned Into 'Horror Show.'"

The misinformation in the article started with the idea that people with diabetes "smear" their drops of blood onto thin plastic strips to get a blood sugar reading from their machine. If I did that, my reading would of course be inaccurate. I likened this image to a horror show (hence the headline). The article went on to say that people with diabetes inject insulin into their muscle, which is untrue (the target is the layer of fat just below the skin so insulin can be absorbed effectively). Then it said that losing consciousness was the "worst scenario" a person with diabetes could experience if their blood sugar went too low. In reality, a coma or even death can result, which most people would argue is an even worse scenario than losing consciousness.

I thought that was it. The newspaper's readership had been misinformed through a front-page article, so I wrote a letter that clarified the details of diabetes management and pointed the finger—mistakenly, as it turned out—at the author of the article. When my letter ran, however, it was accompanied by an editor's note saying that the then president of the Langley branch of the CDA, Judi Lee-Richards, had approved the article. Apparently, it wasn't the paper that didn't get the facts straight. It was the CDA.

The damage was already done. The Langley population, through mass media, was misinformed about diabetes. It was my first lesson in distortion and misinformation in the media and how it can lead to public perceptions that are incorrect. Instead of promoting diabetes awareness, as per the CDA's mandate as a nonprofit organization, the association promoted ignorance and misinformation by clearing an inaccurate article.

Nonprofits are not always burdened by the politics and underfunding that the CDA faces. Recently a perfect issue surfaced, and the CDA revealed its inability to affect any change and its toothless stance on issues that concern those with diabetes.

Human insulin has been on the market for some years. Before this, animal insulin from pigs and cows (known as pork insulin and beef insulin) was used extensively. Some people with diabetes had adverse reactions to the human insulin, mostly resulting from their inability to tell when they were having an insulin reaction. Animal insulin also affects the body differently than human insulin.

Lilly, one of the companies that makes insulin, decided not to offer animal insulin anymore in Canada. Many people who relied on these animal insulin products complained, but to no avail. The decision had been made and animal insulin was no longer carried in the pharmacies. Lilly said they would gradually phase out animal insulin, but it didn't work that way.

I use human insulin, so the change did not personally affect my treatment, but many others who relied on animal insulin were left hanging. Because they wish to continue with animal insulin, they procure it by any means necessary, even if that means buying it from sources in Europe who still use animal insulin widely. Who provides the insulin in Europe? You guessed it—Lilly.

What has the CDA done in the face of this issue? Nothing. Even with prominent physicians, diabetes groups and many individuals involved in demanding an answer, the CDA is speechless on this issue and hesitant to be involved. Their response to this pressing issue shows that the CDA is unable to advocate for people with diabetes at a time when many of us need it most. Maybe it's not part of the budget.

Camps Potlatch and Winfield

Being part of the CDA youth group enabled me to learn about diabetes camp, which is arguably the best reason for the CDA's existstence. There was a time they stopped camp for liability reasons because someone got hurt or had a reaction, but to my knowledge, camp for kids is alive and well.

I enjoyed being a camp counsellor at two CDA camps that are both stories in themselves. Potlatch was a risk to the CDA, but it was fun. Luckily for us, the CDA did not realize that it was too remote, off the coast of Britannia Beach in B.C.'s Howe Sound. Winfield was a Lion's camp outside of Kamloops, B.C., and was considerably safer.

Imagine thousands of cedar trees and the occasional bear visit. That was what Camp Potlatch was like. In the middle of nowhere, nestled in a pure, pristine wilderness. No television, and the only communication being a radio to the mainland.

The ferry comes into the harbour and drops off the kids and doesn't come back for the duration of the camp. The kids are stuck there at Camp Potlatch until the end. As counsellors, we came out on a boat before the ferry to endure the training. The camp was run by the CDA, but it was open to children without diabetes as well as those who have the condition. The same was true for the counsellors.

I was impressed that children without diabetes were matched up with those who had diabetes, as were the counsellors. It became quite a learning experience for all involved. Each child challenged the boundaries set upon him or her by diabetes and had fun doing it.

I remember waking up and making our way to the lodge where we'd all collectively take our insulin and test our blood sugar. This experience amplified the fact that a child was not alone—others also had this chronic condition and were enjoying camp with everybody else. Diabetes was only a small part of the whole camp experience. As a counsellor, I realized that I was a role model of sorts. Someone to look up to, at a time when looking up to someone was important.

I remember listening to gangsta rap up in the middle of nowhere. We went on a camp trip into the wilderness. I can remember camping there out in the boonies, our packs weighty, though we hardly complained. We found heaven in a canoe, rowing off to a secluded island, alone and wild, into the broken mist and finally away from what had limited us for years, finding solace in a stone and the trees that bent the world in a moment.

This was eternity here, in the calm songs sung by someone who knew them, in the crackling of a fire burning, attending the Potlatch campfire. We raided cabins in the warm summer night, itching for a glimpse of the sorry souls who were nestled in the temporary sanctuary of their sleeping bags. This was heaven—

forgetting that we even had diabetes at all.

I was paired up with a counsellor nicknamed "Ice," who did not have diabetes. By pairing a counsellor who had diabetes with a partner who didn't, everyone could be sure that things went smoothly. There were only two times I can think of that there was actually a scare.

One involved a girl having an insulin reaction at a Potlatch campfire. She had "brittle" diabetes, which meant unpredictable swings in blood sugar. Snack had been too late for her. It was a waiting game—it always is with a low blood sugar. I remember this incident purely because of the reactions of the medical "professionals." Yes, there were nurses and a doctor there to make sure everyone was taking their insulin and eating a bit more than usual.

When the girl at the campfire had her insulin reaction, the nurses freaked out. When she was brought in unconscious by Ice, it was a crazy sight. They treated her with glucose gel, sticking it into her mouth and rubbing it into her gums and inside cheeks so the sugar would absorb into her bloodstream. Ironically, it was the girl herself who was the least fazed by the whole event, happy to finally recover after receiving a glucagon shot.

This girl woke up dribbling sugary gel all over and feeling like an idiot for not recognizing that she was getting low and putting everyone through so much trouble. Almost everybody there breathed a sigh of relief; of course, it wasn't her fault.

A nurse exclaimed how she was going to quit her job right there and then. In the heat of the situation I suppose everything is up for grabs, though I think the medical staff could have been more empathetic. It could be that the textbook explanation of low and high blood sugar is a different thing altogether than experiencing the reality of hypoglycemia. Why do you think it's nicknamed insulin "shock"?

If a medical professional cannot handle one episode of hypoglycemia, perhaps some more medical training might be in order. This nurse was clearly unprepared to deal with the rigours of diabetes, yet the CDA was legally required to have doctors and nurses on staff to make sure stuff like this didn't happen.

Another incident occurred when Ice and I led a group of campers river walking. Navigating rapids and walking up on the stones was actually quite fun. We had packed a lunch and walkie-talkie radios for safety, as any day hikers had to do.

The idea was to hike up until we found a bridge that had a trail to take us back to camp on land. Unfortunately, we passed under the bridge and never found the trail. We weren't alarmed, and we kept hiking higher and higher up the river. We kept thinking the miraculous log bridge would appear just beyond the next set of rocks. We couldn't find the bridge and it was getting late. We figured it was possible it had been knocked out during a storm or when the river floods during winter. Eventually, we had to radio for help.

The same medical people were hiking up with us, including the nurse who already wanted to quit. They again blew the problem out of proportion. We were halfway down the river when people from camp came with blankets and the like, but we were completely fine. We made it all the way and it was an adventure.

Potlatch must have become too much of a liability with stuff like that happening. That was the last time the CDA used the site. This was unfortunate, because Potlatch was one of the greatest campsites I have been to—there are many memories that I am fortunate enough to have because of Potlatch.

Winfield is a B.C. Lions camp up near Kelowna, B.C. The CDA clearly chose it because it was much safer than Potlatch. In other words, it wasn't as remote from medical facilities and civilization.

My eight-year-old nephew attended Winfield, and it was great to be a counsellor and have him there. He also has type 1 diabetes. I remember the emergency snack boxes set up around camp so that campers could chow down if they felt they were having an insulin reaction. Camp tends to lower the blood sugar because of all the excitement and activity.

There were actual stations strategically placed around the

campground to deal with low blood sugars. If a camper became too low, he or she would seek out one of the red wooden boxes in which there was a peanut butter and jelly sandwich (which we nicknamed PBSes). As a counsellor, I can attest that campers did get low and needed PBSes to bring their blood sugar back into the normal range. These odd emergency rations were replaced every day. The snacks at bedtime were increased, blood sugar levels were measured meticulously and insulin dosages were carefully tracked to make sure everybody stayed with the program. All in all, the CDA was playing it much safer at Winfield.

Camp contributes to any child's self-worth. A group spirit can be fostered, as well as confidence, security and independence. Of course even more interesting is adventure. Both camps were excellent experiences and I learned so much. I'd recommend summer camp to anyone. It nurtures a sense of accomplishment to survive the wilderness—and it's fun.

At camp, I met many people who had diabetes with different lives and ways to treat their condition. I found I was not alone and that I could help people through setting some sort of example. I also found that diabetes is a different thing to different people. For example, people differ in the way they recognize they are having an insulin reaction. These were intimate moments shared in the darkness among boys with type 1 diabetes. Such revelations were never shared in a focus group.

Strangely, as I think back, some of the most inexpressible experiences of my life were experiences had at camp. I will never forget how kids appreciated just being in a different time zone from their parents. Just being there playing games, organizing cabin raids, partnering with a cool camp counsellor called Ice, and canoeing in the middle of nowhere made it all worthwhile, somehow.

We were pushed to the boundaries but made it back without a serious mishap. It felt good knowing we could do it, that we'd taken a risk and that we'd beaten the odds.

I have not been back to experience any other CDA camps, which are now held at another location altogether. Camp is one of the only things that made the CDA worth it for me.

Juvenile Diabetes Research Foundation (JDRF)

It was the Juvenile Diabetes Research Foundation (JDRF) that announced the 1990s as the "decade of the cure." We've now passed the year 2000 and the decade of the cure has elapsed. Nonprofits promise cures every five years or so in the name of fundraising; those who are living with diabetes and its related complications often cling to false hopes perpetuated by nonprofits.

I have participated in the "Walk for the Cure," an annual fundraising event run by the JDRF. The JDRF doesn't do as much in the way of providing information as the Canadian Diabetes A ssociation does, but as an organization it seems more focused on fundraising for research.

JDRF promised a cure, however, and they haven't delivered it. Whether it was a ridiculously optimistic marketing ploy to drum up more funding for diabetes or a reason to remain hopeful that a cure for diabetes would come in the 1990s, the "decade of the cure" it wasn't.

Promising a Cure

Diabetes management is an extremely profitable industry. Pharmaceutical companies make billions of dollars in profit from supplying insulin, syringes and blood test strips to an increasing market, not to mention nonprofit organizations that make fundraising their focus. One of the latest conspiracy theories I've heard of is that diabetes has become "too profitable to cure." Now, the same organizations are focusing on diabetes management, which seems to have eclipsed the search for a cure. Research has given us advanced and faster blood glucose monitoring, thinner syringes, plastic (rather than glass) syringes, quicker-acting insulin, synthetic human insulin and the insulin pump, among other things.

It's clear that people with diabetes are a captive audience to a growing market. If scientists found a cure for diabetes tomorrow, these companies (and nonprofit organizations) would suffer a tremendous blow to their business. What is most prudent for businesses involved, then, is a focus on diabetes management.

Conspiracy theories aside, I am sure a cure will come for diabetes. It might be in the form of a vaccine for people genetically at risk for developing diabetes. It might be through transplanting Islet cells or some other cure currently unknown, but don't hold your breath. (I've tried it but after a while your face turns blue and people will start to yell at you to stop it.)

While there could be a cure just around the corner, it is more immediately vital that we treat people better now—and I'm not talking about diabetes management. Looking to the future for a cure or for better ways to manage diabetes will not help us treat people today where they need it the most.

The wildly optimistic pronouncements from nonprofits and news media are often aimed at people who can fund diabetes research, not people who are living with diabetes. We need to focus instead on what can be done now to change our attitude towards those who have diabetes; to help us recognize that there are people with this condition, and that it is serious illness that is not easily explained.

Chapter 10
Demystifying Science and Medicine

Like a Cookbook: Science and Conventional Medicine

Diabetes demands many changes of people, requiring lifestyle, diet and scheduling modifications. A study by Elaine Sullivan touches upon the idea of change in patients with diabetes. Because diabetes is self-managed, decisions regarding insulin, diet and exercise must be juggled by the patients themselves.

Indeed, those with diabetes are:

> ...expected to make multiple (complex) changes at the same time...(which) involve understanding the effect of exercise patterns, medications, and dietary intake level on blood glucose. The process is not static; change in one or all of the behaviours may not entirely correct a problem. [29]

Doctors and nurses often expect these changes to show an immediately beneficial result, rather than teaching a person to understand the complexity of the physiological changes in their bodies and incorporate these changes into their own decisions regarding self-management.

Health providers, furthermore "tended to oversimplify diabetes self-management, not recognizing that this task is a very complex and demanding challenge." [30]

To be fair, health providers are busy and don't necessarily have the time to spend hours explaining the complexities of diabetes with each patient. But that does not excuse doctors from the requirement to help people learn about their illness. Doctors speak from a privileged position in a society that sees them as authoritative. Doctors' orders often trump a patient's own understanding of his or her condition, even if the patient has been living with diabetes for years. This may not always be for the best, however, since diabetes is different for everyone, and in many cases it is the person with diabetes who is most attuned to the physiological effects of the condition. When it comes to treatment, therefore, what works for the individual is the key—the doctor, importantly, doesn't necessarily have the latest treatment guidelines or your best interests at heart.

I believe that medicine, informed by the scientific method, has to take the back burner to a person with diabetes' own experience. The restrictions currently imposed on someone with diabetes by doctors who think they are doing something good can be ridiculous; such doctors tend to act as if diabetes was an acute condition, like a broken arm that can be easily managed and cured. Many medical professionals, sadly, do not deal with the condition on an individual level, and it is left up to the person with diabetes to find suitable professionals to treat it properly.

If I demanded that a person without diabetes stop eating anything that contained sugar for the rest of life, he or she would laugh. However, I was told never to eat anything with sugar in it, even though sugars are now considered a meal choice for people living with diabetes. People with diabetes can work food that contains sugar into their meal plan, because the diet focus is now more on carbohydrates. So why are there all those people making money off outdated "diabetic" cookbooks? It could be these are the same people who are exploiting the diabetes market by selling glucose tablets and glucose gel, when a packet of sugar or some honey will do just as well as these specialized and pricey alternatives.

Listen to what the medical team tells you, but remember it is not the word of God. You must take control of your own body. Easier said than done, understandably.

Aldous Huxley said that:

...science is just like a cookery book, with an orthodox theory of cooking that nobody's allowed to question, and a list of recipes that mustn't be added to except by special permission from the head cook...[31]

More people should be questioning science because it shapes how we view the world, especially with regard to medicine and the treatment of diabetes.

Conventional medicine has been criticized on many levels. Rosalind Coward, in her book *The Whole Truth: The Myth of Alternative Medicine*, argues that conventional medicine:

• Endangers health, considering profit more important than people
• Treats diseases and symptoms rather than people
• Perpetuates inhumanity
• Induces unnecessary suffering
• Rarely attends to feelings or emotions
• Does not allow for patient control over treatment

Ironically, many of these points run opposite to the Hippocratic oath. People are starting to realize that some of the "major events of life—birth, illness, and death—have been horrendously mismanaged in a society where status and profit (predominate)." [32] This viewpoint is increasing as people turn to alternative medicine, or traditional medicines, but why did these criticisms surface? Why does the practice of medicine limit itself to scientific modes of thinking? Clearly, the foundation of modern medicine began with science.

Science and Myth as the Foundation of Medicine

If we are cured of disease, we explain the matter by saying a pill or a serum did it—as if that were to say anything at all... We believe that somewhere behind the pills...there are experts who understand whatever else there is to understand. We know they are experts, because, after all, they talk like experts and besides possess degrees, licenses, titles and certificates. Are we any better off than the savage who believes his fever has been cured because an evil spirit has been driven out of his system? [33]

Theodore Roszak, in his book *The Making of a Counter-Culture*, raises a salient point about doctors and pharmacists. Why do we put so much trust in pharmaceutical companies? Is it because we believe in a myth of magic pills and concoctions? Or do we believe—consciously or otherwise—that a doctor's prescription will ultimately cure us?

Knowledge is intimately based on human perceptions of the world. These are in turn framed by norms, social codes and values borrowed from religion, myth, science and tradition. These social, cultural and historical contexts are often overlooked when considering medical knowledge and science. We are less prone to question something taken out of context.

Medicine relies on the scientific method, which is considered objective (through separating the subjective, personal feelings by examining only illnesses) and reductionist (by studying the part, for example the pancreas, an assumption is made about the whole body). Over the past century, the scientific system of thought has proliferated, becoming, as Morris Berman writes, "a hostile glare, a scorching ball of fire that, as Dali tried to suggest, even melts clocks in an arid desert landscape." [34]

Science represents legitimate knowledge in our society. To call your work scientific is to baptize it with a mythical standard of accuracy and objectivity that goes unquestioned. Did you ever wonder why they dress some poor guy up in a white lab coat and give him a clipboard to advertise products? Because he looks like a scientist when he's like that. People trust him because of the costume he's wearing. Dress the same guy up in jeans and a T-shirt and you probably won't think he was a scientist (just the millionaire owner of a dot com company).

Science is also obsessed with the concept of measurement. In the West, as David Bohm points out, measurement plays a key role in the way we see our worldview and ourselves. It was Isaac Newton who said "I have measured, that is enough," [35] but though Newton and Rene Descartes' dualism have contributed to this prevailing worldview, it originated in the ideas of Protagoras in ancient Greece, who said "Man is the measure of all things."

Measuring certainly isn't enough. Finding out what my Hemoglobin A1c is gives me a clearer picture of my glucose control over time. It does not suggest that my behaviour has been deficient, or that I have somehow transgressed against the medical establishment (I haven't "adhered" or "complied" with my diabetes regimen). Nor does a simple reading on a console tell me what life is all about.

Surely we can salvage medicine, which has been elevated to the status of a religion for many involved in the system, from the obsession with measurement.

The East, however, recognizes that not everything can be measured, and that the:

Immeasurable (i.e., that which cannot be named, described, or understood through any form of reason) is regarded as the primary reality... Whereas to Western society...measure...is the very essence of reality, or at least the key to this essence, in the East measure has now come to be regarded commonly as being in some way false and deceitful...in the West, society has mainly emphasized the development of science and technology (dependent on measure) while in the East, the main emphasis has gone to religion and philosophy (which are directed ultimately toward the immeasurable). [36]

Morris Berman, in *The Reenchantment of the World*, highlights the immeasurable, which is beyond the purvey of science, focusing purely on the measurable, we fall into a trap of reductionism.

There are so many things science can't explain, and perhaps never will. But there are still people who believe that if something is touched by science, it is knowledge—as if science says it's truth, it becomes truth, like some sort of Midas touch turning everything to gold. According to the Dalai Lama:

> By replacing religion as the final source of knowledge in popular estimation, science begins to look a bit like another religion in itself. With this comes the danger of blind faith in its principles and a corresponding intolerance of alternate views on the part of some of its adherents. [37]

Fundamentalist scientists believe that science is the only way to obtain knowledge, which denies the existence and/or validity of differing forms of knowledge.

The noted quantum physicist Werner Heisenberg introduced the idea that reality cannot be known apart from the knower. In other words, the information known as "reality" cannot be separated from the process that happens in your brain and nervous system, or from the environment. This theory also renews the idea of interconnectedness with the environment, running contrary to the scientific ideal of objectivity and controlled experiments with impartial observers. This just means that a doctor can't stay out of the process. With diabetes, even if the doctor remains emotionally unattached and follows the conventional medicine party line, they're still intimately connected with what's going on around them. In fact, things even change by their presence and power.

It's almost as if the science of physics has come full circle and finally realized that experiments cannot be separated from the context of the person carrying them out. Heisenberg's theories raise many questions about the claims to objectivity and the non-participatory nature of science. Science can be said to be subjective, or dependent on the researchers as they participate in the experiment.

This isn't surprising. It's quite clear that those professing objectivity in science are the ones choosing the statistics to support their claims. Major pharmaceutical companies have the resources to hire truckloads of research assistants that will prove "objectively" through scientific studies that smoking is good for you or that big trucks pollute less than small cars.

Not many scientists want to admit science has a mythical dimension, or that the fine line between objectivity and subjectivity is an illusion.

Joseph Campbell, the pre-eminent mythology scholar, called this the "edge," or the "interface between what can be known and what is never to be discovered because it is a mystery that transcends all human research." [38] Campbell believed that science and mythology do not conflict at all; that science is "breaking through now into the mystery dimensions," and that it cannot explain everything.

In relation to diabetes, and more broadly Western medicine, other ways to obtain knowledge besides science are just as valid. Science is not the only beacon of truth and knowledge there is. It's not objective. It's subjective and participatory.

In relation to diabetes, however, medical professionals claim to know what a person with diabetes is supposed to do to control their condition. Medical science and the experimentation on dogs led to the creation of insulin. Billions have been spent on scientific diabetes research to no avail. In focusing only on science, the holistic approach to treating a chronic illness today and into the future has been considered unimportant. In the obsessive focus on clinics and experiments, the person has been lost in the shuffle.

Surrender to Medical Technology

Neil Postman, in his influential book *Technopoly*, laments the surrender of culture to technology. Part of this is the surrender of medicine to technology; in other words, an increasing reliance on machines to replace the role of doctor. According to Postman, doctors are particularly eager to perform surgery on patients in American hospitals, despite less of a reliance on technology in European hospitals. He says that:

American doctors use far more X-rays per patient than do doctors in other countries. In one review of the extent of X-ray use, a radiologist discovered cases in which fifty to one hundred X-rays had been taken of a single patient when five would have been sufficient. [39]

What does this mean? Why are American doctors particularly zealous with technology and surgery? Money is part of the reason, but it also has to do with liability issues. The patient often demands to see the X-ray, so a physician's recommendations might not be taken. Technology is a double-edged sword.

Lynn Payer, in *Medicine and Culture*, describes the mythical dimension of Western medicine:

> The once seemingly limitless lands gave rise to a spirit that anything was possible if only the natural environment...could be conquered. Disease could also be conquered, but only by aggressively ferreting it out diagnostically and just as aggressively treating it, preferably by taking something out rather than adding something to increase the resistance. [40]

Postman considers the invention of the stethoscope to be one of the first technologies to distance patients from physicians. It essentially transformed medical practice—a doctor could no longer simply rely on a wealth of precedents and treatments. Their own experience was secondary to a new piece of machinery.

Stanley Reiser, in his book *Medicine and the Reign of Technology*, likens the stethoscope to the effects of the printing press on Western culture. The concepts of objectivity and detachment are implicit in his writing. Reiser believes that a physician could "move away from involvement with the patient's experiences" to a supposedly "objective" position. [41] Postman suggests that the stethoscope promoted the ideas that medicine was about disease—not the patient—and that technology was more reliable than either the patient's or physician's experience or beliefs. By subordinating the process to an X-ray, CAT scan, ultrasound or even a Hemoglobin A1c, the physician distances herself from the patient and from her own judgment.

Unfortunately, the physician is placed in an awkward situation if a patient wants results. With the risk of malpractice suits over their heads, especially in the United States where such suits are more common, doctors rely heavily on the technology even if the patient doesn't need the test.

Postman's main arguments about the influence of technology in medicine can be summed up in three main points. Technology:

1. Is not a neutral element in the practice of medicine. Doctors don't only use technology but are used by it.
2. Creates its own imperatives and creates a wide-ranging social system to reinforce such imperatives.
3. Changes the practice of medicine by redefining what doctors are, redirecting attention and changing how they view patients and illness. [42]

Expectations are placed on a doctor to act a certain way. We expect a doctor to perform within a social setting. As Joshua Meyrowitz observes in his book *No Sense, No Place*, we expect a doctor to appear:

Confident, concerned, patient and professional—and slightly superior. We expect a waitress to be efficient, respectful, and non-intrusive. And we demand these differences in "character" even if the waitress is a student earning her way through medical school. [43]

These "roles" are not simply masks that are slipped on and off; they are "personalities we become attached to." When we play a given role, it becomes real not only to the audience, but also to ourselves.

These expectations become part of how a doctor is mythologized—seen as something more than human and someone who is authoritative. In reality, doctors are people too. They may have gone to medical school and recited the Hippocratic oath and learned how to conduct open-heart surgery, but this does not make them superhuman. And it certainly does not make them the ones to have control over your diabetes. Indeed, only you can control your diabetes.

Doctors have skills that enable them to practice medicine. They aren't far off from the mythological healer who would perform rituals to scare away evil spirits—medicine's just acquired a sense of superiority as it borrows from science golden legitimacy, and a full pharmacy of medications.

One could almost say, as Meyrowitz does, that access to information is putting a dent in the almighty practice of medicine. He says that:

> Citizens are constantly seeking information on their "rights" and looking for protection from potential encroachments by high status people, big business or government. And the general trend toward "self-help care," the feminist critique of the medical establishment, the return of lay midwifery, and the rise of "alternative birthing centers" suggest the demystification of the once almighty role of the doctor. 44

Ultimately, diabetes management is not something that should be placed solely in the hands of a physician. It must be the patient who takes responsibility for weighing the advice of medical professionals and acting to manage the disease. Because diabetes has not been cured and can only be crudely controlled with insulin, blame should not be placed on the patient if therapy fails or if complications develop. And just as doctors play certain roles to fulfill their job, a person with diabetes needs to find a doctor who helps him or her live a life of wellness.

Shifting the Focus

Suzanne Johnson, in the *Pediatric Psychology Handbook*, raises another issue concerning medicine, which shifts the focus from patient to medical practitioner. She writes that "in contrast to the wealth of information available on patients' behaviour, there is remarkably little on health care providers' behaviour." [45] This fact is seriously disturbing. It indicates yet another bias on the part of those observing—the other side of the microscope could be the source of many difficulties people with diabetes face.

Johnson further points out that "studies suggest that inappropriate treatment recommendations and inaccurate diabetes knowledge imported by ignorant providers may be responsible for some patients' poor glycemic control." [46] This argument is a persuasive one. Is it the student's fault for not learning if they don't understand the teacher? Is it the student's fault for not learning if the teacher is misinformed? Often, it is a family physician, having to be knowledgeable in myriad areas of medicine, who is the primary information resource for those with diabetes. Telling a person with diabetes that they should try to stay normal is not enough. Medical professionals need to be more informed, and people with diabetes need to demand sufficient treatment for a chronic condition.

Access to information is a serious problem, especially for rural communities. If you live in a small town and happen to be diagnosed with diabetes, it's going to be difficult to keep a pulse on the developments in the diabetes field. This is still true even though the Internet has improved access to diabetes information.

Deb Butterfield writes of her experience with a doctor, illustrating that the person with diabetes sometimes knows more than the medical professionals.

> I had been living in my diabetic body for 24 hours a day, 365 days a year, for 24 years. That was 210,240 hours. If I had worked that many hours in a 40-hour-per-week job, I would have 106 years of experience. Yet, as was often the case, the doctor dismissed me as a layperson and

assumed power of attorney over my decisions. It was a typical example of a chronic illness being cared for in a medical system designed to take care of short-term illness and trauma. [47]

The person who is living with diabetes is the expert on their condition. A doctor should be there to guide, not police or take control.

Suzanne Johnson also thinks, justifiably, that the term "compliance," which is used in much research to describe the "extent to which a person's behaviour (in terms of taking medications, following diets or executing lifestyle changes) coincides with medical or health advice," [48] devalues a patient's own control over his or her condition and places the physician in a role of authority. This point is crucial in dealing with what is a chronic condition. The call for "adherence" is much better, as it "connotes a willingness on the patient's part to follow the physician's recommendations." This point illustrates again how important language is in shaping our conception of illness.

It's not surprising that "adolescents with IDDM (insulin-dependent diabetes mellitus) are known to be less adherent than their younger counterparts." [49] This makes sense given that adolescence already involves enough lifestyle and bodily changes without throwing diabetes into the mix. There is also an increased risk for eating disorders and depression among children with diabetes, something that should not be overlooked.

Adherence and blood sugar control are not interchangeable—there is no consistent link between patient adherence and blood sugar control. A patient may be following a prescription religiously, but blood sugars can still, almost inexplicably, bounce. The HbA1c is not a measurement of behaviour, but a measurement of health status.

Professionals, then, must take a much more holistic approach and view all of the characteristics that make up a human being's complex experience if they want the best chance of success with their treatment.

Treatment is acceptable when it considers a person with diabetes as a whole. People are more complex than a chronic medical condition and shouldn't be labelled as such. People are also emotional and spiritual beings. Historical, cultural and social contexts must play a part because diabetes affects all these levels. Family and social situations are important too. Patients should be allowed to be in charge of their condition, sitting in the director's chair when it comes to defining the best goals of treatment.

Natural and Holistic Therapies

Holistic medicine may be one of the only "…humane alternative(s) to an overly technical, disease-oriented, impersonal medical system." [50]

Holistic therapy is coming of age and there's no end to the books and supplements that are presented as crucial components of diabetes therapy. People are looking beyond insulin.

I borrowed a book from the diabetes group that I attend. All kinds of supplements are recommended for deficiencies and complications surrounding diabetes. Alpha lipoic acid (which may improve peripheral nerve function impaired by neuropathy) and fenugreek (a plant that lowers blood sugar) are just two of the substances extolled. Other plants that may lower blood sugar include dandelions, licorice and ginseng. Physicians continue to scoff at natural therapies, and indeed it is difficult to separate the hype from the actual facts about any given substance. Taking extra substances can affect blood sugar, so a physician should be involved at some level. Ask around and do research about what is recommended and what the risks are. Listen to what people say about the subject.

I cannot make any specific therapy recommendations in this book, though I do know people with diabetes who take supplements with religious devotion, convinced that they are inhibiting certain complications and improving their overall health. If it works for you, that's great.

With complicated lives full of endless choices and information overload, we seem to have less control over what's happening on all levels—individually, within society and worldwide. But of course, much of what we witness, whether it be on the television news reports or through the local newspaper, is filtered and edited, offering a distorted view of the reality of life. The bad news reigns because it's out of the ordinary, not because humanity is all bad.

The holistic health movement offers a way out of this chaotic world by placing control over the whole person in the hands of the individual. The whole, essentially, becomes the focus, rather than conventional medicine's focus on parts. Indeed, I have always found it odd that modern medicine is specialized into different fragments—it seems that you could visit a podiatrist (foot specialist), an ophthalmologist (eye specialist) and an endocrinologist (endocrine system—and diabetes—specialist) and be pulled in all directions with different therapies. Where is the patient with a focus on all these bodily organs? The holistic health movement offers a way out of this problem of fragmentation, but it also brings up issues of its own.

How can this "perfection" of wholeness be reached? With regard to a person with diabetes, it is possible that he or she is blamed for not being a "whole" individual, that contracting diabetes was the result of some sort of imbalance.

Much of holistic therapies suggest that we must be obsessed with our health, so much so that we can't even tell if we're actually healthy. If we are constantly counting carbohydrates, measuring food portions, exercising, testing blood sugars, taking vitamin and herb supplements, and analyzing the state of our health from minute to minute, things can quickly get out of hand and become issues of quality of life.

Maybe that's the point—everyone has an ailment of some sort, an imbalance or neurosis in life that could be worked on. It's not hard to imagine a person with diabetes feeling as though they need to run in marathons to prove to the world that they're healthy and fit to a society obsessed with health.

Which begs the question: Are those who are not "whole" somehow lacking? What if you have diabetes and you're blind? Does that mean you can never be a whole individual? The reality is that as humans we do not have absolute mastery over our health. We cannot prevent diabetes from occurring any more than we can deny our own mortality.

Aboriginal peoples recognize the importance of a holistic approach to wellness. Dr. L. Gilchrist, suggesting Aboriginal peoples should rediscover their natural heritage, says:

> We abdicate responsibility of our bodies to the Western medical industry. As a people we are hugely doctored, medicated, operated on and irradiated, and yet we have the highest illness and mortality rates... The importance of the integration of natural and holistic methods into a complementary medical model of illness treatment, health risk reduction and prevention, cannot be overestimated when we consider the many implications of modern life for Aboriginal peoples. [51]

Wellness is possible even in the face of diabetes, through integrating natural and holistic methods that are part of Aboriginal traditions.

Holistic Therapies

Some holistic therapies include:
- Homeopathy (stimulating the body defenses with tiny doses of substances that would cause disease symptoms in larger amounts)
- Aromatherapy (essential oils are distilled from plants or herbs and then inhaled, bathed, or used in massage)
- Ayurveda (suggesting disease as an imbalance of movement, structure and metabolism that needs to be treated with diet, herbs and yoga)
- Acupuncture (insertion of needles into pressure points on the body, thus releasing tension)
- Chiropractic (the spine is the key to health and it needs to be manipulated back into shape)
- Kinesiology (building up muscle strength through exercise)

Holism is not a movement in itself, because there is no uniform set of holistic therapies, as in herbal medicine.

That being said, many holistic therapies share in common certain principles. These are set out convincingly in Kristine Alster's book *The Holistic Health Movement*. I've summarized then elaborated on eight of these principles below. They are useful for this discussion as they relate to a chronic condition such as diabetes. [52]

1. A person is more than the sum of his or her parts. Conventional medicine tends to treat patients as "cases, diseases, symptoms or problems. This kind of care is de-humanizing: the client is being considered as a thing, not a person."

While reductionism shouldn't be used as a form of therapy, it often is. Even the separate specialties of holistic medicine can have a narrow focus. If you had a neck problem, for instance, a chiropractor might diagnose a back problem and treat it, while a massage therapist might diagnose tense muscles and treat those. A person is more than a broken down car that needs a

---

- Herbal medicine (plants are used to treat illness and enhance physical functions)
- Shiatsu massage
- Macrobiotics or other lifestyle diets
- Megavitamin therapy
- Crystal therapy
- Spiritual healing
- Folk remedies (traditional medicine)

While this is not an exhaustive list of holistic therapies, it gives an indication of the wide spectrum of therapies considered "alternative" by conventional medicine. It might be worthwhile to note that many of these therapies are being adopted by physicians; acupuncture, for instance, is often conducted by a conventional medical doctor.

mechanic, whether therapies are conventional or holistic. That is to say that if you put a whole bunch of body parts together, you won't have a living, breathing, emotional and spiritual being. You'd have Frankenstein.

2. *There is no mind/body split.* Descartes' dualism is a misconception, because people are intimately connected as a whole. The mind cannot exist without the body and vice versa. Descartes said, "I think therefore I am," which seems to me to be quite a selfish statement. Our thinking is based largely on this selfish notion that I exist because I think.

3. *Good health is more than physical well-being.* Health is balancing physical, mental and spiritual aspects of a person in harmony with the environment. Just because my body functions, it doesn't mean that I'm perfectly healthy. And just because I suffer from a condition such as diabetes, it doesn't mean that I can't achieve a state of well-being.

4. *Because illness signals an "imbalance," it can be a learning experience, providing an opportunity to change a lifestyle.* This may be more true for people with type 2 diabetes who need to adjust their diet and take some pills. Indeed, any illness survived is a learning experience, and the day-to-day existence with diabetes is certainly that, as this book illustrates.

5. *Prevention of illness and the maintenance of health are more important than treating disease.* Not enough conventional medicine is preventative. It is a fact that all diabetes supplies should be handed out free of charge to those who treat their condition. It's clear that managing diabetes closely will help prevent complications later in life. In other words, governments will save a lot of money if they supply people with diabetes supplies rather than wait until they end up in the hospital. An ongoing program of diabetes monitoring would be useful to ensure that diabetes-related hospitalizations would decrease.

6. *Although conventional medical care is useful, and sometimes necessary, self-care is preferable.* With diabetes, self-care is not optional. It's a Do-It-Yourself approach to diabetes that is the reality of my existence. I can't give conventional medicine any credit when it comes to continuing chronic diabetes care. The initial diagnosis, however, did scare my parents and me into "compliance" with a restrictive diet and a stifling schedule that did not fit on the first days of diagnosis.

7. *Caring is a significant component of the healing process.* It's not too surprising that people heal faster when people care. Seniors live longer even when they have a pet cat or dog—the human touch is that much more important.

8. *Unorthodox techniques and therapies often work, even if their efficacy has not been confirmed by scientific testing. Low technology, non-invasive, "natural" remedies are especially desirable.* If it works, it shouldn't need a thousand clinical trials and doctors boycotting it because it hasn't been tested on rats. I can't help but think of the medicinal marijuana argument. It has healing properties for people suffering from disease, so why not legalize it and not criticize it? Alcohol does so much more damage to society through drunk driving and its nature as a depressant. Nicotine is probably the most addictive substance on Earth. Yet even marijuana hasn't been adequately tested for its possible healing properties. Beyond the THC that makes you stoned, there are other ingredients that are obviously at work here.

Similarly, therapies that work should be used, even if they haven't confirmed by scientific testing. Of course, taking a realistic and informed approach to such therapies is important. I remember a naturopath telling me he could cure my diabetes.

"CURE it?" I asked, thinking he was some sort of spiritual healer, "I won't have to inject any insulin at all?"

"Well, no, not exactly. I can lower your requirement for insulin."

In other words, a "cure" is different things to different people, and if all it means is a reduction in insulin, who really cares? I have to take the injection either way.

The medical community has been accused of being close-minded about people. How could this be improved?

A first step might be a willingness to consider that the scientific method is not the only way to approach the practice of medicine. The body is more complex than merely a sum of its parts and cannot always be measured by instruments. People are more than symptoms and more than a collection of bodily organs.

Health involves the body's constituent parts working together as a unified whole. Wellness is not perfect, it is a condition that is acceptable. It is peculiar that modern medicine does not see a chronic condition as acceptable. It cannot because disease is something to be fought, destroyed and treated acutely. Preventative medicine is another area that is often neglected by modern medicine. If the disease exists, steps are taken to destroy it through pills or surgery.

Chronic means forever. A chronic condition may be best treated by a combination of modern medicine and holistic therapies—a merging of Eastern and Western philosophies.

When considering the whole, we become more human. When reducing something to its component parts, we run the risk of losing perspective. The observer is necessarily a part of the subject observed. With regard to diabetes, it is imperative that the medical community recognizes the importance of considering someone as a whole person. Not merely a "diabetic," but a living, breathing human being with a chronic condition.

The aim for a person with diabetes and the team of practitioners that assists her can be balance, harmony and well-being, including body, mind, emotions and spiritual needs.

Drafting Your Team

> The burden of living with diabetes is often grossly under-estimated by even the doctors and nurses directly involved. [53]

There is no better person to make such a statement about doctors and nurses than Deb Butterfield. In her book *Showdown With Diabetes*, Butterfield chronicles the trials and tribulations of having diabetes. She writes about undergoing agonizing complications, then requiring combined pancreas and kidney transplants.

To counteract the alienation inherent in being treated as a disease rather than a person, a person with diabetes must be allowed choice in his or her own treatment. Empowering those with diabetes to be active players—in fact, the directors—of their treatments should be a priority. This sense of participation is vital. Those with a chronic condition can be healthy. Despite the blood tests, the occasional low blood sugar, the insulin injections and eating time, the person with diabetes is not always conscious that he has a chronic condition. To focus solely on his disease is to deny that he is a functioning human being within society, not merely a "diabetic," but a writer, a firefighter, an engineer or a Nobel Prize winner.

Similarly, those with diabetes should realize that they could be perpetuating this cycle by putting their least appealing foot forward by introducing themselves as a "diabetic." Consider the well-meaning person with diabetes who, in an interview, introduces herself as "Jane, the diabetic" certainly, such a revelation is brave, but considering so much relies on first impressions and that Human Resources is quite likely to discriminate against her on the basis of a medical condition, she needs to weigh the options. If there's any indication from the popularity of drug testing employees before they are hired, companies still discriminate on the basis of a medical condition. This is not the best way to start a discussion, unless it's with a medical professional about treatment.

Wellness means adaptation. It means the ability to consider oneself as a whole person, despite resignation, self-denial and helplessness fostered by cultural beliefs of having to adjust or fail. Being a whole person does not mean isolating oneself. JoAnn LeMaistre, in the book *After the Diagnosis: From Crisis to Personal Renewal for Patients with Chronic Illness*, says "there is no more effective way to isolate yourself than to continually appear self-sufficient, denying any need for help or comfort from others." [54]

To find a doctor that you trust and respect the first time around would be a considerable stoke of luck. Often a family physician is inadequate to deal with specialized diabetes issues. Sometimes they are willing to learn and listen, but in most cases, it's better to seek out a trustworthy doctor who specializes in endocrinology.

Patient responsibilities:
• Avoid burnout by not trying to learn everything at once.
• Ask questions and accept only full answers.
• Manage your health by understanding how your body works and how it is affected by diabetes.
• If the doctor-patient relationship isn't working, find another doctor.
• Report negligence or improper conduct.

Medical professional responsibilities:
• Remove moral judgements from treatment of diabetes.
• Attempt to maintain a supportive relationship.
• Realize that diabetes isn't only about medical care, but about nutrition, exercise, emotions and a host of other complexities.
• Treat patients as whole human beings, not "diabetics."
• Answer questions, but be patient while patient is trying to cope with information overload, especially at the time of diagnosis.
• Don't expect a person with diabetes to change everything in their lifestyle at once.

The most important member of the team is you, because you make most of the treatment decisions day to day and take control of diabetes. All the other members of the team make recommendations based on their experience and can help if you need guidance, but ultimately, treatment is up to you, and following treatment recommendations is a choice.

Conclusion
LOOKING ON THE BRIGHT SIDE OF LIFE

I do not think that suffering is good for you. I never have thought that and I never will. I think it can be, if you take it right, but that is all. If I could, I would get rid of my diabetes faster than the speed of light. I think it is a perversion of Christianity to want suffering. [55]

Teresa Mclean's words ring true. Suffering is not good for you. Who would want to live with diabetes? It's an uphill battle, as is life. However deep the suffering, don't forget that you aren't alone. Everybody suffers to some degree. It's how we react to suffering that brings out our humanity towards others.

When I was seventeen, I decided I would create an art project relating to diabetes, much to the annoyance of my parents. I took each 1/2 cc syringe I used, which was two a day at the time, and saved them until I had amassed an impressive collection. I later spelled out the word "ALIVE" by sticking used syringes into the wall. It was a way to convince myself that I was indeed surviving and could literally spell life out of insulin syringes. Despite being a biological hazard in my bedroom, it helped me through a rough time. I encourage anyone to express feelings through art as catharsis.

Long ago at the Canadian Diabetes Association office, a man brought in his own art project. A woman who worked there suggested photographing it for the front cover of a magazine, though it was horrifying. It was a baby rattle, made up of syringes and with insulin bottles for eyes and dripping glue tears. It expressed much of the profound sadness associated with diabetes. Apparently the man had just recently been diagnosed, having his lifestyle dramatically changed to support a chronic condition. It was never photographed or published, to my knowledge.

Inevitably, diabetes is a burden on the body and the brain. As the experience of diabetes is different from person to person, it seems no one plan for diet, insulin and exercise can offer a definite solution for each individual. Tackling diabetes is a process of continually learning and evolving. One has to find what works and take science, medical prescriptions and holistic medicine with a dose of critical awareness.

Pretending diabetes isn't there won't make it go away. Calling insulin a cure is an exaggeration of a nonetheless significant discovery in medicine. People with diabetes are all around, though some employers attempt to exclude them from workplaces, governments attempt to restrict their licenses and many people go on believing misconceptions.

What You Can Do
Here are a few suggestions to make your life with diabetes more bearable:
- Join a support group or create one yourself.
- Join a church group or youth group.
- If you need help, ask for it.
- Write in a diary about your life and your ideas.
- Become an expert—learn everything your can about diabetes (but it's all right to go at your own pace).
- Talk to people about diabetes and try to dispel the misconceptions about diabetes.
- Keep in touch with your doctor, but most importantly, find a doctor you like ask them questions.
- Include your diabetes team in your treatment
- Write a book.

It cannot be stressed enough that people *have* this condition; they are not the condition itself. To label people as a medical condition denies their diverse personal qualities. I am indeed not a diabetic. I am first and foremost a student of life. I am a writer. I am a swimmer. I am a guitar player. There is a subjective entity in this body coming to terms with diabetes. I doubt I ever will, but I can try. Living with a chronic condition should make anyone proud of being alive and living life to the fullest.

Thank You

I sincerely hope reading this book has helped you under-stand diabetes a little bit more. If you have been newly diag-nosed, welcome to the club, and my heart goes out to you. You are the reason I wrote this book.

If you're a medical professional, please don't sue me, because these are predominantly my personal ideas and opinions (except, of course, where I quoted others).

If you're someone who picked up this book wanting to learn more about diabetes for the sake of a family member or for interest, thank you, too.

There's a person behind the chronic condition that needs you to understand.

Appendix 1
Glossary

Alpha Cells: Type of cells in the pancreas responsible for producing the hormone glucagon.

Banting, Frederick: Discoverer of insulin in 1920. A maverick doctor who was apparently a poor scholar who took a very good idea and ran with it, despite the criticism he received.

Best, Charles H.: Co-discoverer of insulin at the University of Toronto. He founded the Canadian Diabetes Association in 1953 as support group for people with diabetes. It has since grown into something entirely different.

Beta Cells: The cells that make insulin, which are found in the Islets of Langerhans in the pancreas.

Blood Sugar/Blood Glucose: Measurement of the amount of sugar in the bloodstream at any given time. The ideal range is 4 to 8 millimoles per litre. People with diabetes refer to this as "high" (hyperglycemia) or "low" (hypoglycemia).

Blood Sugar/Blood Glucose Meter: A hand-held machine that tests blood sugar levels. Pricking a finger with a lancet of some sort enables a drop of blood to be placed on a strip that is inserted into the meter. The meter then reads the drop with light and displays the blood sugar level.

Calories: Units that represent the amount of energy provided by food. Primary sources of calories are carbohydrate, protein and fat. Calories that are consumed and not used as energy are usually stored as fat.

Canadian Diabetes Association (CDA): A nonprofit organization founded in 1953 by Charles Best, whose mission (should they decide to accept it) was to promote the health of Canadians through diabetes research, education, services and advocacy.

Carbohydrate: A source of calories. Carbohydrates come from sugar (simple carbohydrate) and starch (complex carbohydrate.) Examples of complex carbohydrates are pasta, bread and beans. Carbohydrates are broken down into glucose and raise blood sugar levels eventually.

Cholesterol: A yucky fatty substance that the body actually creates in the liver to build cell walls and make vitamins and hormones. Eating too many animal products and saturated fats can lead to this substance collecting along the inside walls of blood vessels. This can lead to a heart attack or stroke.

Counteregulatory Hormones (also called Stress Hormones): Hormones like glucagon, cortisol, growth hormone and adrenaline, which are released during stressful situations. The liver releases glucose and cells release fatty acids during stress for extra energy. Ironically, this stress can lead to more stress over higher blood sugar levels and ketoacidosis.

Diabetes Mellitus: A chronic (lifelong) condition in which the body cannot produce insulin or properly use the insulin it does produce, resulting in high blood sugar levels. The term comes from the Greek words *diabetes,* meaning "passing through," or "siphon;" and *mellitus* meaning "honey-like," or sweet, in reference to the sweet taste of a person with diabetes' urine. *See Insulin-dependent, Non-insulin-dependent and Gestational diabetes for different types.*

Diabetes Control and Complications Trial (DCCT): Conclusive proof that controlling blood sugar levels reduces the risk of diabetes complications, but people with diabetes knew that before 1993, when the DCCT was reported. It was a ten-year study by the National Institutes of Health that cost approximately $200 million U.S. Over 1,400 people with type 1 diabetes followed conventional therapy (two injections a day) or intensive therapy (multiple injections or insulin pump). Despite the gain of intensive therapy, the people in this category had more episodes of low blood sugar and gained more weight. Some diabetes advocates suggested the money should have gone to find a cure, not for diabetes management studies.

Diabetic: An arguably archaic term for a person with diabetes. I am not diabetic. I prefer to be called a "person with diabetes." I am a person before I am a medical condition.

Endocrinology: The study of the endocrine glands, including the pancreas. Most diabetes specialists study this discipline.

Fats: The most concentrated source of calories in the diet. Saturated fats are found primarily in animal products. Unsaturated fats mainly come from plants and can be monounsaturated (olive or canola oil) or polyunsaturated (corn and other oils). Excessive fat, especially saturated fat, can cause elevated blood cholesterol, increasing the risk of heart attack and stroke.

Gestational Diabetes: Diabetes that occurs during pregnancy. It shows up in 3 to 5 percent of pregnancies and disappears after the baby is born. Women who experience gestational diabetes have a higher risk of developing other forms of diabetes later in life, as does the baby.

Glucose: A simple sugar. Complex carbohydrates such as bread, pasta, cereal and fruits are eventually broken down into simple sugars that the body uses for energy or stores as fat. Insulin reduces glucose levels in the blood.

Glucagon: A hormone produced by the alpha cells in the pancreas that increases blood sugar. Glucagon releases glycogen stored in the liver in the event of a really low blood sugar.

Glycogen: The bodily storage form for carbohydrates (glucose) found in the liver and muscles.

Glycosuria: The presence of glucose in the urine.

Hemoglobin A1c (HbA1c) : A blood test that measures overall blood glucose level control. Good to get at least twice a year.

Holistic Approach: A way of thinking that includes the whole individual, rather than focusing on a part of the individual.

Hyperglycemia: The big medical term for high blood sugar. Occurs as a result of an insulin dosage that is too low, inactivity or eating too much food. Major symptoms include excessive hunger and thirst, frequent urination and fatigue.

Hypoglycemia: The big medical term for low blood sugar. Occurs as a result of an insulin dosage, which is too high, exercise, stress or too little food. Major symptoms include excessive hunger, sweating, shakiness, palpitations, confusion and disorientation.

Impaired Glucose Tolerance (IGT): Blood sugar is high, but not high enough for diabetes diagnosis. Commonly referred to as "borderline diabetes" which is misleading, but people with IGT are at an increased risk for developing diabetes.

Insulin: A hormone secreted by the pancreas that enables sugar to enter blood cells, thus producing energy. Insulin injection is required for people with IDDM to survive.

Insulin-dependent Diabetes Mellitus (IDDM): A common name for type 1, or juvenile diabetes. Occurs in about 10 percent of the diabetes population. It usually occurs in people under 30 years of age, and is caused when the immune system attacks the beta cells of the pancreas and the pancreas can no longer produce insulin. The pancreas does not produce any insulin, so it must be injected. Heredity, stress, viruses or autoimmune dysfunction could be factors, but medical professionals haven't figured out the cause yet. (It should be noted that some people with type 2 diabetes also become insulin-dependent, but all people with type 1 diabetes are.)

Insulin Pump: A machine that injects insulin automatically and regularly into the body.

Insulin Reaction: *See Hypoglycemia.*

Insulin Resistance: The most common cause of type 2 diabetes, where the body does not respond to insulin properly.

Islets of Langerhans: The insulin and glucagon producing cells of the pancreas. Named after Paul Langerhans who discovered them.

Ketoacidosis (Diabetic Coma): A condition caused by a lack of insulin or severely high stress hormones. Ketones are present in the urine and blood sugar levels are high and the body tries to consume fat, muscle and vital organs for energy by the digestive system. This causes a buildup of acid in the blood, which is serious and fatal if not treated immediately.

Ketones: Acids produced when the body burns fat for fuel. This occurs when there is a lack of insulin or when there are severely high stress hormones.

Lispro Insulin (also known as Humalog): A clear, rapid-acting insulin that begins to work in 5 to 15 minutes, peaks in 1 hour, and has a duration of 3 to 4 hours. Insulin pumps ususually pump lispro insulin in very small doses over long periods of time, thereby helping stabilize blood sugars.

Metabolism: Process, including all physical and chemical changes occurring in the body, in which food is broken down and used to provide energy necessary for maintenance and growth.

mg/dl: Milligrams per deciliter. One way to measure blood sugar levels. The other is millimoles per litre (mm/l), depending if you're using the metric or imperial system.

Nephropathy: Renal (kidney) disease.

Neuropathy: Any disease of or associated with the nerves, usually causing numbness.

Non-insulin-dependent Diabetes Mellitus (NIDDM): A common name for type 2, or adult onset, diabetes, although some people with type 2 do become insulin-dependent. Occurs in about 90 percent of the diabetes population. Understandably, there is a problem with the terms. A person with non-insulin-dependent diabetes does not have the same condition as a person with insulin-dependent diabetes, though both suffer from diabetes. Non-insulin-dependent diabetes usually occurs in people over 40 years of age, but is currently an epidemic among aboriginal peoples, developing in younger people. Most with NIDDM are insulin resistant, but some simply cannot produce enough insulin to meet their bodies' needs, and others have a combination of these problems. Many people with NIDDM control the disease through diet and exercise, but some must also take oral medications or even insulin injections.

NPH Insulin (also known as Lente, N or L): Cloudy, intermediate-acting insulins that begin to work 1 to 3 hours after injection, peak in 6 to 12 hours, and last from 18 to 24 hours.

Ophthalmologist: An eye specialist who can check out your eyes and prevent nasty developments. Should check your eyes at least once a year.

Pancreas: The organ of the body that produces insulin as well as performing other digestive functions. It is located just behind the stomach. With IDDM, the pancreas does not produce any insulin, so it must be injected. With NIDDM, the pancreas produces some insulin, but not enough to sustain a normal blood sugar.

Podiatrist: A doctor who specializes in the treatment of the feet and disorders related to the feet.

Protein: A source of calories in the diet. Protein provides the body with material for building blood cells, body tissue, hormones and other important substances. It is found in meats, eggs, milk and certain vegetables and starches.

Regular Insulin (also known as R or Toronto): A clear, short-acting insulin. It begins to work 1 hour after injection, peaks in 2 to 4 hours, and has a duration of 6 to 8 hours.

Retinopathy: Disease of the eye specifically concerning the retina.

Sugar: A form of carbohydrate that provides calories and raises blood glucose levels. There are a variety of sugars, such as white, brown, confectioner's, invert and raw. Fructose, lactose, sucrose, maltose, dextrose, glucose, honey, corn syrup, molasses and sorghum are also sugars. When reading a label, just look for the "ose."

Sugar Substitutes: Sweeteners used in place of sugar. Note that some sugar substitutes have calories and will affect blood glucose levels, such as fructose (a sugar, but often used in "sugar free" products) and sugar alcohols like sorbitol and mannitol. Others have very few calories and will not affect blood glucose levels, such as saccharin, acesulfame K and aspartame (NutraSweet).

Type 1 Diabetes: *See Insulin-dependent Diabetes.*

Type 2 Diabetes: *See Non-insulin-dependent Diabetes.*

Ultralente Insulin (also known as U): A cloudy, long-acting insulin that begins to work 4 to 6 hours after injection and has a minimal peak effect, which is helpful for some people. It lasts from 24 to 28 hours.

Urine Test: The definition of humiliation, which measures substances in the urine, including sugar. This was how doctors used to assess blood sugar control in the pre-blood-sugar-meter era. Unfortunately, it does not offer an accurate reading, as it measures a person's blood sugar level many hours before the test. Ketones can be detected this way.

Appendix 2
Top Ten Misconceptions About Diabetes

Ever since I was diagnosed with diabetes I've heard all kinds of misconceptions about diabetes. These appear most frequently as questions directed at me after the bomb is dropped—that is, after I tell someone I have diabetes.

Sometimes it's much easier to hide the fact of diabetes in the closet than it is to declare to everyone you meet that you have it. Why? Because the following misconceptions are so much a part of people's psyche. It leads to discrimination against those with diabetes.

Think carefully about the following misconceptions and be prepared to challenge them.

1. Eating too much sugar causes diabetes. Genetics are the biggest cause of diabetes. If it's in your family, you're more likely to get it.

Rest assured that chocolate bars do not cause diabetes. Nobody really knows exactly what causes diabetes yet. What is known, however, is that the destruction of the insulin-producing cells (Islets of Langerhans) occurs as an immune system response. What is not known is why.

2. All people with diabetes have to take shots. Ninety percent of those with diabetes have non-insulin-dependent diabetes, which means they treat it with pills, diet and exercise. Ten percent of those with diabetes have insulin-dependent diabetes. These people, including myself, have to take shots.

It is a fact that people with type 2 diabetes, most of whom are not insulin-dependent, receive much of the media attention, and this only serves to exclude those people who don't fall into the high-risk demographic for type 2 diabetes. Each time I pick up the paper or find an article in a magazine I hope it will be different—but too often it's an article framed as a warning for those over age 40 to be tested for diabetes, or warning that people may already have diabetes and not even know it.

The last time I checked, I have diabetes, and no, I'm not over the age of 40. Such articles have an affect on public perceptions about diabetes. People might remark that those with type 1 diabetes are "too young" to have diabetes. This is just one of the misperceptions perpetuated by nonprofits such as the Canadian Diabetes Association (CDA), the media and the rumour mill.

3. Diabetes is not a serious illness like cancer or AIDS. Many people underestimate the seriousness of diabetes. Diabetes is a leading cause of death by disease in North America. Some 2.25 million Canadians and 16 million Americans have diabetes. In 1998, 750,000 people had AIDS, and 8 million had cancer in the U.S.

Much funding, however, goes to diseases with a larger public profile, diseases that capture the public's attention. Indeed, both AIDS and cancer are horrible diseases that have touched many lives. Diabetes, however, has touched even more.

4. Those with diabetes cannot eat sugar. Sugars are considered part of a balanced diet, along with proteins, breads, fruit, vegetables and milk. The food groups are important when planning a healthy diet, whether or not you suffer from diabetes.

No foods are forbidden for people who have diabetes. It's actually the carbohydrates that raise blood sugar, and sugar is only one type of carbohydrate.

5. Those with insulin-dependent diabetes have a choice of treatments. Insulin is the only widely available treatment for insulin-dependent diabetes and has been for the last 75 years. Insulin pumps offer an alternative to syringes, though they are expensive.

6. People with diabetes can't play sports or exercise. I played basketball through high school. I was no Michael Jordan, but I had fun. Many people with diabetes are professional athletes. People with diabetes are involved in a wide variety of sport activities from rugby to skating. There is even an athletes' association for those with diabetes, which holds conferences about diabetes management issues and keeping fit.

Many athletes use the pump because it offers more flexibility when training. Athletes are less likely to want a big dose of insulin sitting in their system while they're training for the triathlon.

7. People with diabetes are overweight and old. Some people with diabetes are old and obese. People, however, come in all shapes and sizes, and it would be unwise to assume that all those with diabetes fit one body type.

Those with type 1 diabetes are generally no more obese than the average North American. If you met me on the street you probably would not know I had diabetes.

This misconception is attributable to type 2 diabetes, which often affects those who are obese and old.

8. Diabetes has been cured. Insulin is a cure. Insulin is not a cure for diabetes. Diabetes has not been cured yet. Insulin can merely control the illness, not stop it, therefore, diabetes is a chronic affliction that, in some cases, requires constant injections of insulin.

Insulin allows diabetes management, and without it, people with diabetes wouldn't be here.

9. Insulin shots are injected into a vein, like a drug addict shoots up.
Insulin is not injected into the bloodstream via a vein. It is
injected into the fat tissue just below the layer of skin. A fold of
flesh is pinched and the shot is injected into the fold. This allows
for a slower absorption than would happen if injected directly
into the blood.

The insulin pump works in much the same way, however it
releases tiny doses of insulin over a long time, thereby approxi-
mating the normal functioning of the pancreas. Each meal is
covered by a "bolus" , given through the pump, of lispro (short-
acting insulin) that is adjustable, depending upon the carbohydrates consumed at the meal.

10. People with diabetes make poor workers. They get sick all the time.
There is nothing to substantiate this misconception, even
though many employers actively refuse to recruit those with diabetes. This is unfortunate, as it forces people with diabetes to
keep it a secret from their employers, lest they be skipped for
promotions or health coverage.

Appendix 3
Famous People who have (or had) Diabetes
(no distinction made between type 1 or 2)

Piers Anthony, science fiction writer
Jack Benny, actor
Halle Berry, actress
James Cagney, actor
Fran Carpentier, *Parade Magazine* editor
Johnny Cash, musician
Nicola Cavendish, actress
Paul Cezanne, French impressionist painter
David Crosby, musician
Miles Davis, musician
Mama Cass Elliot, musician
Thomas Edison, inventor of the light bulb, telephone and phonograph
Ella Fitzgerald, vocalist
Nusrat Fateh Ali Khan, vocalist
Ernest Hemingway, writer (*The Old Man and the Sea*)
Nicole Johnson, Miss America 1999
BB King, vocalist
Peggy Lee, vocalist
George Lucas, film director
Curtis Mayfield, musician
Mary Tyler Moore, actress
Elvis Presley, "The King"
Mario Puzo, writer (*The Godfather*)

Q Tip , DJ (A Tribe Called Quest)
Anne Rice, writer (*Interview With the Vampire*)
Elizabeth Taylor, actress
Neil Young, musician
H.G. Wells, writer (*The War of the Worlds*)

And many more...

Appendix 4: Millimoles and Milligrams Conversions*

mmol/l = millimoles/litre
mg/dl = milligrams/decilitre

mmo/l	mg/dl	observation
2	35	Really low. Eat sugar.
3	55	Low. Eat sugar.
4	75	Ideal range.
5	90	Ideal range.
6	110	Ideal range.
8	150	Ideal range.
10	180	High.
11	200	Even Higher.
15	270	Uh-oh.
16.5	300	What did I eat?
20	360	That can't be.
22	400	I'm getting thirsty.

*After consulting this chart, please note: There is no such thing as a "bad" blood sugar reading. Blood testing is good as it helps you to control your condition, so pat yourself on the back for doing it at all in the first place.

Appendix 5: Diabetes Information

American Diabetes Association (ADA)
The ADA provides diabetes research, information and advocacy.

1701 North Beauregard Street
Alexandria, Virginia 22311 USA
Phone: 1-888-342-2383
http://www.diabetes.org

Alternative Diabetes
Provides information about alternative approaches to diabetes treatment, such as herbal, dietary and nutritional strategies.

2005 South 91 Street
Omaha, NE 68124 USA
Phone: (402) 393-6391
http://www.alternativediabetes.com

Canadian Diabetes Association (CDA)
Supports diabetes research, education and advocacy.

15 Toronto Street, Suite 800
Toronto, Ontario
M5C 2E3 CANADA
Phone: 1-800-BANTING (1-800-226-8464)
http://www.diabetes.ca

Diabetes UK
Formerly the British Diabetic Association, Diabetes UK works for people with diabetes by funding research, campaigns, and helps people living with diabetes.

10 Queen Anne Street
London W1G 9LH UK
Phone: 020-7323-1531
http://www.diabetes.org.uk

Juvenile Diabetes Reasearch Foundation (JDRF)
Founded by a group of parents of children with diabetes, the JDRF seeks a cure through funding scientific research.

7100 Woodbine Avenue, Suite 311
Markham, Ontario L3R 5J2 CANADA
Phone: 1-877-CURE-JDF
http://www.jdfc.ca

Yahoo
Has a useful listing of Web sites on diabetes.
http://dir.yahoo.com/Health/Diseases_and_Conditions/Diabetes

Joslin Diabetes Center
Established in 1898, an internationally recognized diabetes treatment, research and education institution affiliated with Harvard Medical School.

One Joslin Place
Boston, MA 02215 USA
Phone: 1-800-JOSLIN-1 (1-800-567-5461)
http://www.joslin.harvard.edu

Children With Diabetes

Web site designed to promote understanding of the care and treatment of diabetes, especially in children.

23548 Calabasas Rd, Suite 202
Calabasas, CA 91302 USA
Phone: (805) 492-6530
http://www.childrenwithdiabetes.com

Rick Mendosa's Web Site

Rick Mendosa, a freelance journalist who has diabetes, maintains this directory of diabetes-related Web sites.

238 Coronado Drive
Aptos, CA 95003-4011 USA
Phone: (831) 688-5300
http://www.mendosa.com/diabetes.htm

Diabetes Frequently Asked Questions

http://www.faqs.org/faqs/diabetes

Appendix 6: Selected Bibliography

Alster, Kristine Beyerman (1989) *The Holistic Health Movement*, University of Alabama Press: Tuscaloosa

Beaser, R.S. (1994) *Outsmarting Diabetes: A Dynamic Approach for Reducing the Effects of Insulin-Dependent Diabetes*, Boston: Joslin Diabetes Center

Becker, Howard S. (1963) *Outsiders: Studies in the Sociology of Deviance*, New York: The Free Press

Berger, Peter L., and Thomas Luckmann (1966) *The Social Construction of Reality: A Treatise in the Sociology of Knowledge*, New York: Doubleday

Berman, Morris (1981) *The Reenchantment of the World,* New York: Cornell University Press

Bliss, Michael (1982) *The Discovery of Insulin,* Toronto: McClelland & Stewart.

Bliss, Michael, and Mladen Vranic (1996) *The Discovery of Insulin at the University of Toronto,* Toronto: Thomas Fisher Rare Book Library

Bohm, David (1988) "Postmodern Science and a Postmodern World" in David Ray Griffin (ed.) *The Reenchantment of Science: Postmodern Proposals,* Albany, NY: State University of New York Press

Bohm, David (1980) *Wholeness and the Implicate Order*, London: Routledge & Kegan Paul

Boston Women's Health Collective, The (1976) *Our Bodies, Ourselves: A Book by and for Women*

Butterfield, Deb (1999) *Showdown With Diabetes*, New York: W.W. Norton and Company

Campbell, Joseph, and Bill Moyers (1988) *The Power of Myth*, New York: Doubleday

Corry, David (Summer, 1996) "The Sky's The Limit" in *Diabetes Dialogue*

Coward, Rosalind (1989) *The Whole Truth: The Myth of Alternative Medicine* London: Faber and Faber

Davidson, Mayer B. (April 3, 1998) *Testimony Before the IOM Committee on the NIH Research Priority-Setting Process*

Diabetes Control and Complications Trial Research Group (1993) "The Effect of Intensive treatment of diabetes on the development and progression of Long-term complications in IDDM," *New England Journal of Medicine*, 329, no. 14, p. 977–86

Eliot, Alexander, Joseph Campbell, and Mircea Eliade (1976) *The Universal Myths: Heroes, Gods, Tricksters & Others*, New York: Meridian

Edelwich, Jerry and Archie Brodsky (1998) *Diabetes: Caring for Your Emotions as well as Your Health*, Reading, MA.: Perseus Books

Giroux, Louise (1998) *Taking the Lead: Dancing with Chronic Illness*, Kelowna: Northstone Publishing

Johnson, Suzanne B. and Michael C. Roberts Ed. (1995) "Insulin Dependent Diabetes Mellitus in Childhood" in *Handbook of Pediatric Psychology 2nd Ed.,* New York: Guildford Press

Langley Times (November 4, 1992) "She's In Control"

Langley Times (November 14, 1992) "Diabetes Turned Into 'Horror Show'"

LeMaistre, JoAnn (1995) *After the Diagnosis: From Crisis to Personal Renewal for Patients with Chronic Illness*, Berkeley: Ulysses Press

Mazur, Marcia Levine (1998) "Come fly with me; today, for pilots with insulin-treated, well-controlled diabetes, the sky's the limit" in *Diabetes Forecast*

Mclean, Heather and Barbara Oram (1988) *Living With Diabetes: Personal Stories and Strategies for Coping*, Toronto: University of Toronto Press

Mclean, Theresa (1985) *Metal Jam: The Story of a Diabetic*, New York: St. Martin's Press.

Meyrowitz, Joshua (1985) *No Sense of Place: The Impact of Electronic Media on Social Behaviour,* New York: Oxford University Press

Postman, Neil (1992) *Technopoly*, New York: Vintage.

Raymond, Mike (1992) *The Human Side of Diabetes: Beyond Doctors, Diets & Drugs,* Chicago: Noble Press

Rubin, R.R., Biermann, J. and Toohey, B. (1992) *Psyching Out Diabetes: A Positive Approach to Your Negative Emotions*, Los Angeles: Lowel House

Reiser, Stanley J. (1978) *Medicine & the Reign of Technology,* Cambridge: Cambridge University Press

Roszak, Theodore (1969) *The Making of a Counter-Culture*, New York: Doubleday & Co., Inc.

Sontag, Susan (1978) *Illness as Metaphor*, New York: Straus and Giroux

Starr, Paul (1982) *The Social Transformation of American Medicine*, New York: Basic Books

Endnotes

1. *Health Canada* (1999) "Diabetes in Canada: National Statistics and Opportunities for Improved Surveillance, Prevention and Control, Minister of Health." Many people underesti mate the seriousness of diabetes. Diabetes is a leading cause of death by disease in North America. It is estimated that approximately 18,000 Canadians die as a result of diabetes and its complications like heart and kidney disease, stroke, blindness and amputation each year.

2. Lindner, Laurence (1999) "Eating Right: The facts and myths about diabetes," in the *Washington Post*

3. Butterfield, Deb (1999) *Showdown With Diabetes,* New York: W.W. Norton, p. 20

4. Murray, Christopher J. L. and Alan D. Lopez (1996) Global Health Statistics (from 1990), U.S.: World Health Organization. North America/Europe has approximately 38 million with diabetes; former Socialist economies in Europe have 12 million; India has 18 million; China has 10 million; Latin America and the Caribbean has 11 million each; and Middle East has 13 million; other Asian islands have 13 million; and sub-Saharan Africa has 4 million people with diabetes.

5. *Health Canada* (1999) "Diabetes in Canada," p.15

6. Ibid., p. 30

7. Davidson, Mayer B. (April 3, 1998) *Testimony before the IOM Committee on the NIH Research Priority-Setting Process*

8. Juvenile Diabetes Research Foundation statistics

(*http://www.jdfc.ca*)

9. Bohm, David (1980) *Wholeness and the Implicate Order*, London: Routledge & Kegan Paul, p.20

10. Mclean, Theresa (1985) *Metal Jam: The Story of a Diabetic*, New York: St. Martin's Press, p.53

11. Johnson, Suzanne Bennett "Insulin-Dependent Diabetes Mellitus in Childhood" in Michael C. Roberts (ed.) (1995) *Handbook of Pediatric Psychology, 2nd ed.*, New York: The Guildford Press, p.264

12. American Diabetes Association (1990) Position statement: Hypoglycemia and employment/licensure, *Diabetes Care*, 13, p. 535 & Songer TJ et al. (1989) Employment spectrum of IDDM, *Diabetes Care*, 12, p. 615-622.

13. Frank Tannenbaum and Edwin Lemert first mentioned labelling theory. Tannenbaum had served time in prison as a conscientious objector. He coined the phrase "dramatization of evil" to describe the tendency of authorities to label someone a delinquent with the result of the person internalizing the label. He also thought that "we treat people in terms of the categories into which they are placed rather than in the fullness of their humanity." Tannenbaum, Frank (1938) *Crime and the Community,* New York: Ginn and Company, p.165 Lemert divided labelling process into primary and secondary labelling processes. The first doesn't usually translate into social stigma by law enforcement, because it is undetected or unrecognized as deviant; it is the second labelling process by authorities that can confirm a commitment to antisocial actions, because the deviance has been committed as a result of the label.
Lemert, Edwin M. (1951) *Social Pathology,* New York: McGraw-Hill

14. Shoemaker Donald J., (1996) *Theories of Delinquency, 3rd. ed.: An Examination of Explanations of Delinquent Behaviour*, New York: Oxford University Press, p. 192

15. Becker, Howard S. (1963) *Outsiders: Studies in the Sociology of Deviance,* New York: The Free Press, p.9

16. Wilson, James Q. and Patricia Rachal (1977) "Can the Government Regulate Itself?" *The Public Interest,* 46, p. 3–14 as quoted in Binder, Arnold, Gilbert Geis, Dickson Bruce (1988) *Juvenile Delinquency: Historical, Cultural, and Legal Perspectives,* New York: Macmillan Publishing Co., p.164

17. Mclean, Theresa (1985) *Metal Jam: The Story of a Diabetic*, New York: St. Martin's Press, p.49

18. Howie, Lisa, "Director of Driver Fitness" (December 30, 1998) letter to Michael Twist

19. Butterfield, Deb (1999) *Showdown With Diabetes,* New York: W.W. Norton, p.237

20. Alster, Kristine Beyerman (1989) *The Holistic Health Movement,* University of Alabama Press: Tuscaloosa, p.123

21. Edelwich, Jerry and Archie Brodsky (1998) *Diabetes: Caring for Your Emotions as well as Your Health,* Reading, MA.: Perseus Books, p. 23

22. Ibid., p. 276

23. Butterfield, Deb (1999) *Showdown With Diabetes,* New York: W.W. Norton, p. 163

24. Diabetes Control and Complications Trial Research Group (1993) "The Effect of Intensive treatment of diabetes on the development and progression of Long-term complications in IDDM," *New England Journal of Medicine,* 329, no. 14, p. 977–86

25. Butterfield, Deb (1999) *Showdown With Diabetes,* New York: W.W. Norton, p. 168–169

26. Ibid., p. 51–52

27. Hoover, Joan (1989) in a letter to the National Institutes of Health. Hoover argues that it would "make more sense to spend Federal medical research funds in an effort to eliminate the disease, than on a long range study on how to 'live with it,' and in a manner that diabetic patients themselves say they cannot achieve."

28. Edelwich, Jerry and Archie Brodsky (1998) *Diabetes: Caring for Your Emotions as well as Your Health,* Reading, MA: Perseus Books, p.96

29. Sullivan, Elaine Doherty (Jan/Feb 1998) "Struggling With Behaviour Changes: A Special Case for Clients With Diabetes," *Diabetes Educator*, 24, no. 1, p. 76
30. Ibid., p. 76
31. Huxley, Aldous (1982) *Brave New World*, London: Grafton Books, p. 224
32. Coward, Rosalind (1989) *The Whole Truth: The Myth of Alternative Medicine*, London: Faber and Faber, p. 201
33. Roszak, Theodore (1969) *The Making of a Counter-Culture*, New York: Doubleday & Co., p. 259
34. Berman, Morris (1981) *The Reenchantment of the World*. New York: Cornell University Press, p. 185
35. Ibid., p. 33
36. Ibid., p.22–23
37. Dalai Lama (Tenzin Gyatso) (1999), *Ancient Wisdom, Modern World: Ethics for a New Millennium*, Little, Brown: London, p. 12
38. Campbell, Joseph, and Bill Moyers (1988) *The Power of Myth*, New York: Doubleday, p. 162
39. Postman, Neil (1992) *Technopoly*, New York: Vintage, p. 94–95
40. Payer, Lynn, (1988) *Medicine and Culture: Varieties of Treatments in the U.S., England, West Germany and France*, New York: Penguin Books, p. 127, as quoted in Neil Postman (1992) *Technopoly*, New York: Vintage, p. 95–96
41. Reiser, Stanley (1978) *Medicine and the Reign of Technology*, Cambridge: Cambridge University Press, as quoted in Neil Postman (1992) *Technopoly*, New York: Vintage, p. 99
42. Postman, Neil (1992) *Technopoly*, New York: Vintage, p. 105
43. Meyrowitz, Joshua (1985) *No Sense of Place: The Impact of Electronic Media on Social Behaviour*, New York: Oxford University Press, p. 31
44. Ibid., p. 167. For a more in-depth account of the feminist revolt against the traditionally male medical establishment, see The Boston Women's Health Collective (1976) *Our Bodies, Ourselves: A Book By and for Women*, New York: Simon and Schuster. For a discussion on the rise and fall of the

authority of doctors, see Paul Starr (1982) *The Social Transformation of American Medicine*, New York: Basic Books

45. Johnson, Suzanne Bennett "Insulin-Dependent Diabetes Mellitus in Childhood" in Michael C. Roberts (ed.) (1995) *Handbook of Pediatric Psychology, 2nd ed.* New York: The Guildford Press, p. 266

46. Ibid., p. 276

47. Butterfield, Deb (1999) *Showdown With Diabetes,* New York: W.W. Norton, p.126

48. Haynes (1979), p. 2–3 as quoted in Ibid., p. 267

49. Ibid., p. 268

50. Starr, Paul (1982) *The Social Transformation of American Medicine,* Basic Books: New York, p. 392

51. Gilchrist, Dr. L. (09/01/1998) "Get Back to the Natural," *Windspeaker,* 16, p. 6

52. Alster, Kristine Beyerman (1989) *The Holistic Health Movement*, University of Alabama Press: Tuscaloosa, p. 56

53. Butterfield, Deb (1999) *Showdown With Diabetes,* New York: W.W. Norton, Foreward, xi

54. LeMaistre, JoAnn (1995) *After The Diagnosis: From Crisis to Personal Renewal for Patients with Chronic Illness,* Berkeley: Ulysses Press

55. Mclean, Theresa. (1985) *Metal Jam: The Story of a Diabetic,* New York: St. Martin's Press, p. 203

Index

Holistic medicine, 59, 143
Holistic therapies, 132-135, 138
Hormones, 19, 59, 147, 150, 152
Hospital, 27-38
Hyperglycemia, 32, 55, 57, 146, 149
Hyperglycemic, 56, 67
Hypoglycemia, 32, 40, 49-50, 57, 81, 83, 115, 146, 149, 150, 168

Injection(s), 12, 15, 19, 21, 32, 33, 38, 46, 50, 53, 58, 60, 61, 62, 63,
        65, 66, 74, 78, 79, 86, 93, 96, 102, 138, 139, 148, 149, 151,
        152, 153, 156, 157
Insulin, 60
Insulin pumps, 65, 151, 156
Insulin therapy, 96-98
Insulin-dependent diabetes, 12, 13, 15, 19, 21, 97, 131, 147, 150, 151,
        153, 155, 156,

Johnson, Suzanne Bennett, 56, 130-131
Juvenile diabetes, 21, 86, 116, 148, 162

Ketoacidosis ("K"), 56, 64, 146, 150

Labels/Labelled, 13, 23, 74, 76-78, 94, 95, 96, 132
Lemert, Edwin, 168
Lispro Insulin, 53, 60, 61, 68, 99, 151

Meyrowitz, Joshua, 128

Needle(s), 31, 32, 34, 35, 36, 65, 79, 80, 91, 92
Non-insulin-dependent diabetes, 19, 21, 147, 151, 153-154

Obesity, 20-21, 22, 68
Oral gel, 50
Oral medications, 151

Pharmaceutical companies, 12, 60, 68, 94, 98, 107, 118, 123, 126
Postman, Neil, 126-128

Rachel, Patricia, 77
Reductionism, 23, 123, 124, 135
Reiser, Stanley, 127
Risk factors for diabetes, 21-22
Roszak, Theodore, 123

Sugar, 15, 19-20, 23-26, 29-34, 36, 40-41, 43-45, 49-68, 70-73, 75,
        81, 85, 88-91, 96-98, 112, 114-117, 121, 131-132, 139, 146-155,
        160
Suicide, 100-101
Sullivan, Elaine 120
Symptoms of diabetes, 20, 56

Travelling, 87-88
Type 1 diabetes, 5, 12-13, 19-21, 70, 75, 80, 85-86, 107, 110,
        116-117, 148, 150, 153, 155-156
Type 2 diabetes, 13, 19-21, 68, 70, 110, 136, 150-151, 153, 155-156
Type 3 diabetes, 19, 21-22

Wellness, 129, 134, 138, 140
Williams, Daryl, 86
Wilson, James, 77
World Health Organization, 13, 167